The Grand Purpose

(Look Internally Versus Externally)

Mark D. Colafranceschi D.C.

Editor: Lisa Mitchell, Meridian, Idaho - White Owl Advising LLC.
Contributors: Lisa Mitchell, Terry P. Welsh, Hannah M. Rahn, David Douthwright
Cover Art: bengs.ibrahim@gmail.com

Lightning source
Ingram Sparks
US and Canada: +1 (855) 99SPARK or (855) 997-7275
International: +44 (0) 845 124 4643

Printed in the United States of America
The Grand Purpose
p. cm.
ISBN EAN 9780692113592
Subject Code:
OCC011000 Body, Mind & Spirit : Healing - General
OCC011020 Body, Mind & Spirit : Healing - Prayer & Spiritual
MED057000 Medical : Neuroscience
MED004000 MED014000 MED060000
FAM000000 SEL026000

First Edition
14 13 12 11 10 / 10 9 8 7 6 5 4 3 2

Dedicated to my father and mother.

"Live Grand with Purpose"
MDC

FOREWORD

We live in a world that is seemingly complex, yet it is simplicity itself that has the answers to most questions that seem to elude us. We come into this world as a Perfect Thought, a Perfect Idea, a Perfect Concept and shortly after our entry, things begin to change.

The human body, the perfection with which we are born, is an amazing instrument of creation and it is continually sending us messages/whispers that most of us interpret as problems when, in reality, they are simply signals encouraging us to pay attention. It is the body talking to us through pain and discomfort because it realizes that it is the easiest way to get our attention. Unfortunately, we have been trained to misinterpret the message to be a problem and therefore we seek treatment for a symptom that need not be treated at all. We then approach healing from a place of fear rather than careful introspection and the consequences of that action, more often than not, create even more significant problems for us.

The Grand Purpose is a book in which Dr. Mark Colafranceschi, DC, helps us understand the myths that abound in the traditional medical model and how to use our own, inner-physician to apply principles in healing as well as other elements of life. Finding success in any facet of life requires an emphasis on personal responsibility and shedding the attachment to being the victim or blaming our negative situation on genetics, luck or chance. Dr. Cola's primary goal is to guide us through the process of discovering true causation rather than merely trying to manage symptoms. From the Buddhist perspective, life is about suffering on the way to wholeness/nirvana. Suffering is the message that we receive to keep us on our path to personal freedom – or not. This philosophy can apply to the many different facets of life: our bodies, our minds, relationships, money, business, addictions, etc. Pain and suffering are merely signals that we receive to make us aware that something needs to change. The degree of suffering is an essential consideration as to the achievement of long-term success.

You will learn in the Grand Purpose that the body innately understands how to fix itself. In the case of a knee injury, the body sends signals requesting aid and the joint begins to swell. When we have a fever, the body cools it off with sweat. We have created entire industries that coach us to believe their intervention is necessary to make us well. If we choose the outside intervention, we then begin a process of treating the symptoms rather than discovering the root cause. Unfortunately, the short-term treatment can, in many cases, lead to additional and more dramatic problems. Dr. Cola will help you to understand why seeking therapy outside yourself may replace true healing with a short-term approach to make us feel better. It's typically fast and easy and makes us feel better with little effort on our part.

The result of this approach could not be any more disturbing. Something needs to change, and the Grand Purpose provides the reason why and the process of how. The examples of our distress are many. The opioid epidemic is a direct cause of our desire to minimize suffering, depression, and anxiety.

The next connection is to our financial, physical and emotional costs. It is abundantly clear that we continue on a path of destruction and the Grand Purpose provides a solution. How we "treat" these and other life-alternating challenge has caused us to become desensitized to the best advice we can get – from our inner physician. Social engineering in this country has given us exactly what we have requested. We asked the medical profession to provide us with the quick fix so that we don't have to be personally accountable, and they provide us precisely that which we seek.

Our belief that the medical system operates in our best interest is a myth and our desire to abdicate our responsibility has resulted in creating a path that leads us (personally and collectively) to our physical and financial long-term suffering.

Sadly, we are a society of NIMBYs (Not In My Back Yard). It's no mystery to many of us that we should change what we put into our bodies if we want to be healthy and happy "long-term" (certainly the donut and Big Gulp or fried chicken and a cold six-pack creates euphoria for our tongue and brain – but not so much for the stomach and head as the toxins do their damage). Quite frankly folks, our systems are broke. There is more demand for organ transplants than we can begin to keep up with. The truth is that we started with perfect organs and somehow, as caretakers, we did not do what we should have (whether knowingly or unknowingly) to keep them happy and healthy. Any good healer would have attempted to educate the patient about the problem as well as how to fix it – had they been given the time and a patient who was willing to alter their behavior to save their precious organ. Unfortunately, that is not how we/the system is wired. The doctor has eight minutes to listen, diagnose and create a treatment plan and the system has coached us to believe that altering our behavior(s) is not the solution. After all, who wants to give up that bag of potato chips?

Is it possible to create a solution to what might be life-altering after an 8-minute conversation? And we want that solution to require little personal effort and certainly not require altering our lifestyle. The model that we have asked the medical profession to create for us finds the cure in the form of a pill that will create a change that oftentimes makes it appear that we have/will improve. That "moment" of improvement most likely will have some form of adverse consequence that we most likely are not aware of when we choose to go down that path. Certainly, we should be personally responsible and understand the impact of our choice to follow the protocol and understand the effects of that decision.

One thing that is certain is that something must change. Sadly, it is not only our "sick-care" system that needs attention. Dr. Cola theorizes that the problem goes beyond our physical health to our financial, emotional and spiritual health.

Alas, it is very easy to get discouraged as we look at the failed health care system and the sick-care system that has replaced it by those that we trusted. There is much to be optimistic about as we seek the grace that begins the healing process. The Grand Purpose can serve as the blueprint for a better life. I have worked with Dr. Cola for almost 10 years, and he has helped me to find and stay on the path to healthy enlightenment. He has helped dispel the myths and reinforced the understanding that the best guide that I have is me. Certainly, there is much to know but, the number of resources available to us via the internet, books, health coaches, etc. are endless. If you genuinely seek the personal freedom that comes with better health (physical or otherwise), it is time for you to take charge of your well-being. I can assure you that no one cares about you more than you. Dr. Cola's revolutionary book, The Grand Purpose, will help you to craft your plan to find that which you seek.

Terry P. Welsh, CFP, CHFC, CLU, AIF
Anchorage Alaska
President Alaska Financial Associates
www.afa-associates.com
May 2018

Terry Welsh is a registered representative with and securities offered through LPL Financial. Member FINRA/SIPC. Investment advice offered through Independent Advisor Alliance, a registered investment adviser and separate entity from LPL Financial.

THE MAP

INTRODUCTION

I remember vividly when I was a young teenager resisting things my father would do for me and/or insist I do. I would confront him and his reply was, *"We are on the same team, I want the best for you."* You and I are on the same team when it comes to the health challenges presented in this book. I am on your team. This book presents sound science; putting together fundamentals to healing that have been ignored and/or misinterpreted. The multiple pieces of the puzzle are explained in detail. As you read this book you may have a concern about contradicting statements and facts. I assure you that this is not the case—keep an open mind and things will be explained. Ideas will connect as the book progresses. The book has been described as radical and provoking—challenging most people's comfort level because it shatters mainstream beliefs.

The goal of this book is to be the last health or self-help book you may need. If you do the work In The Course In Health, The Emotion-Link to Illness change is guaranteed.

SECTION 1

LOOKING FOR HEALTH
IN ALL THE WRONG PLACES

Most people's map or search of healing is based upon external answers to our health problems, along with the belief that our health problems are caused by external means, such as luck, chance, genetics, or the Germ Theory. This germ "theory" will be connected to your relationships, your finances and your health.

With these external causes, the reasoning concludes that the cure must also come from external means. Examples of these external solutions are drugs, vitamins, herbs, homeopathy, acupuncture, crystals, surgery, chiropractic, and the list goes on. This approach is very much confused by the lack of distinction between relief or cure versus healing. Alarming is that facts and science do not support the current approach to healthcare.

This old map focuses and encourages a relinquishment of responsibility. It stresses a need for external treatment to heal and again doesn't differentiate between healing and relief. The right doctors or healer, the magic pharmaceutical drug, or the right pill or herb are the focus. Once the well-intentioned doctor or healer has you believe that you didn't have anything (or very little) to do with your condition, then it is a very easy sell to have you believe that you need something external to heal: drugs, surgery, treatment, etc. The focus is on relief of symptoms while not understanding that the underlying cause is still present.

During the 16th and 17th century the church held a strong position that the earth was the center of the universe, this being called the Geocentric Theory. Dating back to 600 BC, the Bible stated that the world was the center of the universe with the sun rotating around the earth. The church had self-serving reasons for supporting this theory. Any person teaching otherwise was a heretic. Books and teachings from Copernicus and Galileo (among others) were banned. The belief that the earth was the center of the universe amazingly continued throughout the years 1870 - 1920 by the Lutheran Church. The Bible was challenged and corrected by Copernicanism in 1543. This correction was not anti-religion, yet the resistance and attitude were that anyone presenting conflicting views of the Bible or church was bad and wrong. In this case, the church was more concerned about being right than seeking the truth. Today the church is the government and the lobbyists that control it.

Einstein is quoted saying: "The beliefs that have led you to where you are today are not the same as those which will lead you to where you wish to go." This can be interpreted as: if you have a set of beliefs that are not working, you must be open to changing your beliefs to achieve lasting results. The example of the world being the center of the universe was challenged, resisted, and finally accepted.

"The people who are crazy enough to think they can change the world are the ones who do." Apple Computer Inc. 1997

For Copernicus and Galileo, the existing beliefs did not set limits upon their actions and teachings. When presenting their material, challenging the current belief that was incorrect, the system set off to ridicule, shame and punish them. The good people of that time didn't see their ridicule or punishment as such but supported the church in protecting the status quo. Today we have the same well-intentioned posture that attacks challenging beliefs on healthcare. Instead, those who are challenging are called quacks, unscientific, frauds or criminals. This book will test the modern medical system along with natural medical teachings. If your knee-jerk reaction to what is presented is to attack it with emotion versus facts you may be repeating history—similar to those who ridiculed the messengers of the past.

Within the natural and modern medical systems, each delivers opposing approaches to healthcare, yet share the basis or foundation of healthcare by accepting the germ theory. Both the natural medical system and the modern medical health system throw stones at each other, claiming that each is unscientific and dangerous; they both live in thin glass houses (professions). The claim that mainstream medical is unscientific may be a significant hurdle to overcome. If you in your heart believe this, your subconscious will resist because it makes you an outsider, even though it is proven so and must be accepted or embraced. This book sets out many facts showing the lack of scientific basis for modern medicine.

The pattern of building facts around unsupported beliefs happens continually in many professions. Our entire medical system is formed on the germ theory claiming that germs cause illness. Louis Pasteur, followed by many diligent scientists, has proven the connection between the germ (bacteria, virus, fungus, parasites) and illness. There are not many modern medical doctors, natural doctors and/or scientists who would disagree with this connection. However, the critical distinction is whether science can claim that the germ is the cause of the illness or merely a symptom.

If the germ does not cause illness, the reasonable next question is: What causes illness? The answer is complicated and requires explanation. Copernicus and Galileo had to explain how and why the earth was not the center of the universe; they were correct and yet slow at getting their information accepted by the masses. Politics, religion, and money interfered with progression in the 16th and 17th centuries. The map of the universe at that time was obviously incorrect.

The church and many others refused to accept the logical truth. We are creatures of habit who often cannot accept change even with objective facts. Changing beliefs is resisted by fear. The basis of the fear is centered in a belief that we cannot handle the change that comes with the new facts or ideas. Why did so many people not change their incorrect conclusions about the world? Why do many people refuse to change their characterological flaws? We sit back in amazement, wondering why people hold on to erroneous beliefs in light of objective information. Is change impossible for some? Is change painful?

The germ theory and the entire medical foundation are challenged with sound science today. The belief that your health is at the mercy of well-intentioned doctors, insurance policies, luck or genetics is as unsound a belief as the earth being the center of the universe.

CHANGING YOU IS "IN"

In the book *The Death of Ivan Ilyich* by author Leo Tolstoy, the main character reflects back on his life and questions if he has climbed the wrong ladder his entire life; if he has served the wrong purpose; if his beliefs were incorrect.

How do we know if our beliefs and actions that rule our lives are correct and serving? Does holding on to your current belief about money, relationships, and health serve you? Are these beliefs bringing health and happiness? Would you rather be right or happy? A big challenge in this book is questioning your belief about illness: Are germs/bugs the cause of illness? Or genetics, chance or luck? If for your entire life your beliefs on health have been based on incorrect science you may look back and question those beliefs. Ask now if your ladder has been hung on the correct wall.

Understanding what beliefs are and where they come from is a start. How do erroneous beliefs change your life? How do we challenge and correct erroneous beliefs? Changing is the challenge. Change is the process of becoming different. Why we resist change will be examined in depth in this book and workbook.

It is much easier to see others' shortcomings while ignoring our own. When we empathize with their fear, we can then understand the unwillingness to change and then start to apply it to our own lives.

For those who resisted the notion that our world was the center of the universe, it did not change the fact that it is not. When we are given compelling, rational, hard facts which indicate that our healthcare system is not working, or more importantly, that our external focus in addressing our health issues is fundamentally flawed, are you going to resist as many did regarding the center of the universe? Are we willing to stop and address it? When believing or embracing the germ theory or external causes for illness (versus accepting the facts that prove that health and healing is an internal process) are we willing to address it?

The Catholic Church resisted change and was in denial until 1820 when the church allowed another astronomer to prove that the Earth was not the center of the universe. It wasn't until the Catholic Church took responsibility with Pope John Paul II in 1992, admitting that Galileo suffered unjustly at the hands of the Church. The Church praised Galileo's views and behaviors regarding the relationship between science and religion. (Maurice A. Finocchiaro, The Galileo Affair. Berkeley: University of California Press, 1989)

My hope is that it doesn't take another 200 years for people to change their belief in health. The current and past paradigm of health is off course – a misguided belief. Proving that our natural approach and modern medical approach to health is not working is not difficult; moving people to accept this, change, and take responsibility is the real challenge. My hope is that this book will save you time in your process of healing.

The claim that our medical system is failing is based on the fact that illness is increasing. Disease rates increase in spite of the fact that healthcare spending has increased. In any other profession, business or economy, if spending increases and results falter, we call this a failure. Life expectancy has improved over the last hundred years. However, quantity of life and quality of life are not the same thing. There are other factors not related to our healthcare system that have increased our life expectancy. In the last fifty years, our access to a wide variety and selection of nutritious foods from all over the world has aided longevity. Sanitation and our sewer system have a more powerful effect on our health than the medical treatments we worship. You may think that sanitation and our sewer system support the germ theory rhetoric. It doesn't whatsoever. Proper hygiene and education is an internal focus.

The economics of the healthcare failure have not met reality yet. The robbing of Peter to pay Paul is status quo. We continue to believe that our healthcare system just needs more research, time, and money to develop better drugs or treatments. This is simply not true. The belief that there are "magic cures" that our medical system is hiding is ridiculous.

The longer someone holds a belief, the more references they have with that belief, and the harder it is to let go of the old belief. Our society has held onto the same beliefs on healthcare for thousands of years. Similarly, our society had held onto the belief that the world was the center of the universe for thousands of years. It is understandable the challenge we face. Our modern medical system, however, is only 200 years old. It is still in its infancy. Our natural medical system is thousands of years old and both share a fundamental philosophy of the cause and cure of illness. Both incorrectly believe and teach that illness comes from outside and the cure comes from the outside. Our medical system, natural and modern, attempts to intimidate and scare patients into believing they need professional services and specialized prescriptions to overcome their health issues. In marketing it's called "scare care" and it should be illegal.

Very little effort or explanation is given by natural or medical doctors on the distinction between healing and curing and relief. Our modern science of behavioral physiology, behavioral economics, causal relationships and counterintuitive principles that are leading the way in growth and technology have opened the door to challenge what this book sets out to challenge.

When it comes to money, professions, sports, and relationships we are respecting the science that is proving that success does come from an internal-internal approach. Some label it as intrinsic. This intrinsic approach can be explained by the focus being on virtues versus vice. Deeper explanation follows.

When it comes to relationships and finances do we have a distinction between "healing" the relationship or "curing" the relationship or simply giving relief to painful aspects of the relationship? Can we agree that the only sound approach to relationships and finances is healing? Not cures or relief.

Stop for a minute and place yourself in Europe 300 years ago. This renegade claims that the world is not the center of the universe. His premise, his theory, his belief, and his science cannot be easily explained but it's true! Chances are the masses refuse to change their beliefs. Holding onto old beliefs is a common phenomenon when facts disprove the belief at hand. With the world being the "center of the universe," people would have had to defy the church. One would believe they had become an outsider or radical. It's uncomfortable to change beliefs mainly because it creates discomfort. Many may think *who is this arrogant guy to make such a bold radical statement?* If it produces ridicule upon this author I will hold my head high as did those in the past that correctly challenged the mainstream.

"Even when his theory is proven as fact, most refused to believe. In the psychology of human behavior, denialism is a person's choice to deny reality,

as a way to avoid a psychologically uncomfortable truth." Maslin, Janet (4 November 2009).

The denial today is similar if not identical. Illness is an internal manifestation of thoughts, beliefs, and choices. The science supports this. It is stress that leads people to toxic food, overindulgence, inactivity, addiction, worry, fear, sick beliefs, etc. The cause is stress, so we must start there, not in covering up symptoms or naming symptoms. It is uncomfortable to look at change. If your knee-jerk reaction is to look at genetics or accidents as the cause, you are denying yourself of healing. All we can ask is: "how is the denial working for you?"

RELIEF FROM HEALING

All medical and natural treatments can only provide temporary relief (some longer-temporary) from the symptom or condition if the primary cause is not addressed. Does relief care help or cause harm? It is not black and white. Sometimes relief care enables healing to occur if the person addresses the addiction, vice or true cause of the illness. Most times relief care interferes with healing. I claim that any illness is a hidden addiction.

The addictive cause that leads to illness is often ignored while we address only the symptom. Take elevated blood pressure associated with obesity, diabetes or almost any condition. Elevated blood pressure is a symptom. The fact that it can be reduced 100 percent of the time through a waterfast proves that this symptom is reversed when the addictive pattern is eliminated. When the person goes back to their addictive lifestyle the blood pressure elevation returns because the cause of the symptom is not fully addressed. Proximate causes, like diet, are usually focused or blamed on as being the cause of the elevated blood pressure returning. In following and examining the emotional link along with addiction you can separate those who return to normal blood pressure—versus those who require the blood pressure to return—to redirect that person to the addiction. If you accept that illness is a goal-oriented, biological process that has a purpose (and when the blood pressure again elevates while looking at deeper issues) we find remarkable answers. If the common denominator to elevated blood pressure is emotional conflict not resolved—any well-intentioned, restrictive diet will have limiting results. If the common denominator to elevated pressure is emotional conflict and it is addressed, the well-intentioned dietary protocols will have lasting results. Hang on while these claims are explained in detail.

This book will examine relationships, finances and other aspects that affect your health condition. There is not much business for relief care in relationships or marriage counseling. If there was it would look like this: You're in pain with your relationship; you tell your therapist that you are lonely in your relationship and you want extramarital relations to relieve your urge or loneliness; you want to be touched or heard. Your therapist gives you the phone number of other lonely married people. The therapist tells you that you will get relief if you sleep with them. Ah, what a relief!

What about financial pain? You are in deep debt. Your financial guru gets you a refinance loan on your home for more than it's worth; it provides relief but ultimately you can't afford the payment, and you lose your house. Ah, what a relief!

The question of treatments healing a condition arises when someone gets a common cold or bladder infection and takes antibiotics: the symptoms go away. Ah, what a relief!

The argument is that the antibiotic cured the condition. On the surface it appears that way; however, any person aware of physiology and microbiology will challenge this claim or belief. The killing of an opportunistic bug with an antibiotic does nothing to support the immune system that was initially weakened to manifest the condition in the first place. Killing the bacteria may allow for the immune system and the body to maintain homeostasis, but you must ask why the *healthy* person exposed to the same bug did *not* get sick. No different than saying a loan caused your money problems to go away. The loan represents the antibiotics aiding your money problems—the reality is that when loans are used regularly they cause big problems.

Do antibiotics play a role in healthcare ever? Many life-threatening infections have been given relief or a "cure" with the use of antibiotics. Any serious bacterial infection (namely: meningitis, strep throat, and sepsis) can have a positive (relief) outcome with antibiotics. Please understand that the underlying weakened system that allowed for the bacterial meningitis is not helped by the antibiotics. Antibiotics do help the immune system in a way that allows for the natural body processes to heal. However, the focus must be centered on the body requiring healing from the infection. The old way of thinking that supports the germ theory would just say to add more antibiotics. The results are why we have thousands of deaths each year from infections that do not respond to antibiotics. If antibiotics are the answer we should never see any deaths from bacterial infections. Bacterial infections are still the leading cause of death in both eastern and western culture. Why does mainstream and natural medicine refuse to talk about the cause of the bacterial infection? One reason they don't talk about the cause is that they would have to abandon the germ theory. Overprescribing antibiotics is a serious issue in our communities and are contributing to an increase in illness lengths, illness complications, and death. The over-prescription of antibiotics clearly is reflective of the medical system's lack of understanding of the cause and effect of the bacterial overgrowth as it relates to immune function and the grand purpose of illness. The over-prescription of antibiotics parallels the over-prescription of credit cards and loans.

Another example of treatments for healing a condition is found after a knee replacement or hip replacement. There is no question the replacement produces an incredible change. I have often encouraged patients to undergo hip replacement therapy because the pain causes lifestyle problems. I also explain that illness in their joint is like a FIVE alarm fire going on, called inflammation. The hip replacement is not correction by any means; it's like trying to put out a fire and not looking at the cause. The natural gas line is leaking and will most likely cause disaster later on: usually in the form of other inflammatory problems, like heart illness. Kicking the can down the street always requires that you pick it up at some point.

The germ theory flaws addressed in this book in no way deny a connection between illness and germs or sick individuals with their dying cells requiring bacteria, fungus or a virus as a part of the healing process. My strong science-base and respect for the natural principles combined with understanding cause and effect conclude the germ theory is just that - a theory. If the germ theory were a fact we would all be dead! There is no denying the connection between the microbe/

virus and a condition. However, the relationship is similar to making the focus of a murder be on the bullet.

In summary, the infection starts when the balance between bacterial or viral strength and host resistance is upset. In order for a virus, bacteria, fungus or parasite to survive and multiply in a person it must do all of the following: (1) find a way into the person; natural ways to enter include skin (cut) or mucous membrane (throat, eyes, reproductive); unnatural ways to enter are through surgery, needles, etc. (2) The bug needs to find nutrition in the person; usually dead cells, or fungi which thrive on sugar or high salt. (3) Avoid or overcome the person's immune responses; most healthy people's immune system will neutralize the bug (4) Replicate or spread, using host resources: dead or sick cells.

THE FOUNDATION

It is a foolish man who builds his house on sand. Where your financial health, physical health or relationship health is concerned, we must build on rock. Sand is the old way of thinking about health, rock is the correct way. Who is going to tell you the correct way? The advertising and marketing department? The media outlets that are swayed by the advertisers and lobbyists that are their foundation?

If the foundation salesman owns a beach full of sand, he may sell you sand to build your house on. If he owns acres of rock he will sell you rock to build on.

Nothing in the world can take the place of persistence.
Talent will not: nothing is more common than unsuccessful people with talent.
Genius will not: Unrewarded genius is almost a proverb.
Education will not: the world is full of educated derelicts.
Persistence and determination alone are omnipotent.
    -Calvin Coolidge

The beliefs which have led you where you are today are not the same as those which will lead you where you wish to go.
    -Albert Einstein

If a well-intentioned, knowledgeable builder had you build on sand and you believed that sand was a better choice for building versus rock, would this change the integrity of the building? No. If your belief is incorrect it doesn't matter how much persistence and determination you have, you are going to have problems. There is a place for Calvin Coolidge's poem; however, it is helpful only when one is using the correct paradigm or foundation. Hard work and the virtues that surround hard work are what create success. Spending a lot on healthcare doesn't produce health. If you believe that your health is in the hands of doctors, vaccinations, drugs, insurance companies, vitamins, surgery, etc., your healthcare is built on sand. Why not shift to rock? The answer is loaded and complex and will be addressed thoroughly. Who is the author of your belief of where health comes from?

THE ANSWER IS IN THE QUESTION?

If we don't ask the right question, how can we possibly get the correct answer? The question that will resonate throughout this book is asking: what is the cause? (and asking for answers and explanations).

Why do we get sick? What is the purpose of pain? How do my emotions affect my health? Your focus is essential: i.e., is my wrist pain from overuse? My mom and dad had the same condition. How come my other wrist isn't in pain when I use it the same amount? What weakens the ligaments?

What guides our beliefs and decisions on healthcare are the paradigms which we believe governs our health. A paradigm can be compared to a map, which is simply a tool used to get to a destination. The paradigm/map in the 1600s didn't allow for sailing over the horizon. A paradigm/map is either correct (accurate and working) or incorrect (incomplete and or not working). An analogy would be using a map of New York City to navigate Los Angeles. It doesn't matter how persistent, good-looking, charming, rich or dedicated you are, you are not going to reach your destination with the wrong map! If you attempted to reach a destination (i.e., a restaurant in Los Angeles) and were using a map of New York, you would soon realize this futile. After trying the same thing and getting the same unfulfilling results for two or three hours, you might challenge your map (paradigm). If you asked a knowledgeable person on Los Angeles geography, they might tell you your map is incorrect. You would then toss this old map and search for a correct map to get to the destination. The above analogy is painfully evident and elementary. When it comes to our healthcare and the map we use, it is not so obvious to some. Going back to the 1700s when proof that the earth was the center of the universe paradigm was wrong, many still refused to believe the correct map. Why would many refuse to believe?

When we use the existing or old paradigm of health, and we do not achieve our desired outcome, we must question the directions we have been given. The people who do not stop and challenge the map will not achieve health.

The million dollar question this book will answer is why do we continue to use a map (paradigm) for health and happiness that does not work? Many people become hungry for health. Some question the map and look for alternatives, ditching the mainstream medical and going natural. This is not the answer. I call it groundhog's day. It is like a person in an unfulfilling relationship: they realize that the relationship is toxic or abusive; they leave and find a new partner. They soon discover that the new relationship is also toxic – groundhog's day again. Unless you change the map, you get the same thing. I am bold and confident enough to tell you to toss your old map.

If you change from mainstream to natural without shifting your thinking about health you will get the same results. You will be using the same map. Instead of bashing the insensitive medical doctor pushing drugs that produce poor results and toxic side effects, you will instead bash the natural doctor quack that costs a lot and does not get results because he is pushing treatments and supplements that don't get long-term results.

Another way to look at the same pattern is to address the choice of picking food. When we have the choice to stop and eat at McDonald's or Whole Foods, we may choose McDonald's and become sick, fat and depressed. Some may blame McDonald's, and this is the beginning of the stuck-ness. You can't blame McDonald's, you chose it, and it (McDonald's) did precisely what it was supposed to do—make you sick. McDonald's can only do what it is capable of doing; its chemistry is just that. Blaming does not correct anything; your choice as the cause is correct thinking. When you ask yourself why you pick McDonald's instead of Whole Foods you will ultimately conclude that someone who loves themselves will not choose toxic foods repeatedly. The extension of this is that someone who loves themselves will brush and floss their teeth; they will exercise and ultimately select the right partner. Picking your partner then later calling them crazy or abusive is like blaming McDonald's; you may get the judge and jury to agree that it caused you to get fat and have a heart attack but the missing part is that no one forced you.

At present we can blame ill health on many things: tobacco on lung and liver problems; baby powder on ovarian cancer; pharmaceuticals on a lot of illnesses; high fructose corn syrup on fatty liver illness; GMO foods on infertility and the list goes on. We can blame our finances on the government or the economy, our parents, our spouse, kids. We can blame our failed relationships on our exes. We need to change that pattern to get a different result. The profound exercises in the workbook that follows address making lasting, healing changes.

There are many ways to analyze health. One is to look at why people get sick; another is to ask a different question. Why are there people who do not get sick when others around them do? Our modern medical system looks at why people get sick. It diagnoses by way of pathology: it identifies the pathogen as the cause of illness and treats accordingly. This approach may make sense on the surface; however, it is profoundly flawed when addressed with basic deductive reasoning, common sense, and science. The question not asked is: Why did all the other people exposed to the bug *not* become sick? Answering the question and focusing on the healthy turns the natural and modern medical system on its head. The same applies to pills: if they indeed work, why wouldn't they work for everyone? The "cause" of the flu is the bug is similar to saying the cause of someone's death was a bullet. We don't charge the bullet with murder, we charge the person pulling the trigger with murder. Not to argue semantics, but the bullet is just a piece of metal without a person's intervention. The virus is only a simple (non-living) protein.

We apply the same line of questioning with finances and relationships by looking at the principles, foundation, beliefs, and actions of those doing well.

OUR AMAZING BODY

Every second, 7,000,000 (million) of the 25,000,000,000,000 (trillion) red blood cells in your body are removed and replaced by new ones. You create new skin every 30 days, a new skeleton every three months, and a new stomach lining every five days. The molecules of carbon, hydrogen, oxygen, and nitrogen that make up your brain are replaced every year. In fact, 98 percent of all of the atoms that make up your body today did not exist one year ago. Like a river, our bodies are in constant flow; we remove old cells and replace them with fresh ones. With this constant renewal of our physical structures, it would seem that outward changes would be second nature. The truth is, though our bodies are open to change, the interference from our emotions cripples this process. Emotionally, we resist change. Old is comfortable, new is scary. If you were to replace the bricks of your house but didn't have any thought of alternative structures or methods of laying bricks, you would most likely build the same looking house. It is the same with our health.

It is estimated that human beings have approximately 60,000 thoughts a day. It is also estimated that for many of us the majority of these thoughts remain the same from day to day. If we want to experience a different level of health, we must change the bricklaying process as determined by our thoughts, beliefs, and feelings. Otherwise, we will build the same body over and over again. To paraphrase Albert Einstein: Our problems cannot be fixed with the same thoughts and beliefs that were in place when we created them. Again, is the ladder leaning up against the wrong wall?

The preceding facts and our amazing body give us clues as to why so many people heal from conditions. People heal all the time and it's because of internal forces. Change is the miracle.

Sometimes healing is associated with external focus because of the link. If I love to play golf and work hard excelling at the game, I practice and practice. When I improve I say it's because I got the best set of golf clubs or because of my practice. Our conditioning on treatments and medicine creates this pattern of relinquishing our power by attributing healing to external forces.

Most are unaware that 80 percent of back pain resolves on its own. Many people use external modes to aide in back pain relief and during this time when our bodies naturally take care of the pain, we give credit to the chiropractic adjustment or physical therapy. Once someone goes down the path of external treatments the conditioning on the belief becomes harder to correct.

The most drastic healing that takes place within our amazing bodies happens while fasting. Water fasting is not a treatment and in the process, back pain goes away, hypertension drops, and blood sugars normalize. The connection with fasting and changing our thoughts is profound. The connection with fasting and the body's natural correction of illness is profound. We will look at the steps of healing that are required to make 'the fast' healing versus relief…

THE MINDSET

Can you have your cake and eat it too when it comes to health? Can you relax about your diet and exercise and still be healthy? I think you can, and with that answer, there are other factors that will determine this paradox. The "ya buts" are explained in the internal versus external focus. The formula for success with health, relationships, and wealth are the same. Live the principles and processes directed toward internalizing and success is the result. My personal approach is to live clean and do so by wanting to live clean for my Grand Purpose—not just be healthy or fit—rather for something bigger than myself. If through my journey I can make a whole food diet, exercise, and virtues enjoyable and pleasurable, and if through the same work I receive pleasure with my choices then why would I not eat well or exercise?

What if the sound of 'cake' did not bring thoughts of pleasure, rather thoughts of pain? As discussed later, *"The real seat of taste was not the tongue but the mind."* Gandhi

Meth may produce pleasure to someone wanting escape. Cake may produce pleasure to those wanting dopamine release for stress reduction. Trying to get the person to stop wanting the cake without addressing the real reason they want cake will cause failure every time.

The focus of a person in any endeavor makes all the difference. I often ask people if their exercise is internally driven or externally driven. I explain that internally driven exercise is a focus on internal values: the joy of playing in the activity, doing it for enjoyment, passion, connection. The process and time fly by versus the external focus of exercising to lose weight or decrease blood pressure. The physics of the external focus equals long-term failure. The next question is whether your diet is internally driven or externally driven. Most people's focus on food is externally driven and causes frustration and failure. If your food has become a religion, you will fail to heal your condition with an external focus.

The same applies to a person's focus on treatments and taking drugs or supplements. If internally driven we see these modalities facilitating healing. If externally driven: *"fix me doc"* or *"I need to find the right pill"* or new diet is a guaranteed path to failure.

I have studied equally the person who gets sick opposed to the person who doesn't get sick. I have learned more from the person who does not get sick. There are common sense and scientific reasons why people who smoke, don't exercise, etc., live long and productive lives.

The fact that our body does change and heal with incredible purpose and intent shows that we must build on the correct paradigm and not interfere with its innate ability to repair. The next step is addressing the belief that illness is wrong or bad.

The superstitious, magical thinking that doctors, pills, or treatments "heal" must be confronted to be able to change your life. The externally-driven, ego-doctor wants you to believe that the external focus is the way to go. Hence: the need to distinguish between the magic/cure and the miracle/healing. Magic is built on fear or separateness from our belief in healing. This makes the doctor a lot of money—and you sick. It also makes the doc dissatisfied on deep levels.

Pursuing money is very similar to the process of career, business, and jobs. If the focus is money and not on an internal focus of purpose and values of your work, the money then comes with a cost greater than its value. Sometimes the cost of external money chasing is health or relationship illness, while other times the money is fleeting; you obtain it in the external focus and because of that it stays with you temporarily. I believe the attainment and relinquishment of money are directly connected to virtues and serving a Grand Purpose. Have you ever wondered why some attain wealth and then lose it all, or why and how some people obtain wealth and maintain it, even if they have obtained it through dishonest means? These questions—and the answers that follow—parallel perfectly the explanation of your physical health. Keeping in mind that everything is purposeful and that if you attain wealth and lose it, the purpose of losing it is real and meaningful, though it may differ from person to person. For those who look inside to the meaning of losing it, the outcome is rewarding.

For those who obtain wealth through dishonest means and maintain it, there will always be a cost associated with such means. The consequence always affects their health or relationships. Again this is not punishment; it is simply cause and effect. The physics and science of this will be explained, as well as how life is one continuous whole. It is impossible for your finances to not affect your health and relationships, and for your health to not affect your relationships and finances.

The connection between money and relationships, physical health and relationships, physical health and money are all indisputable. It is the stepping back to see how each of these three areas affects the others to be the first step to change.

Understanding the abstract connection between the forces of nature that support and enhance healing—like exercise and diet—while at the same time understanding that healing doesn't require these, takes the further explanation of cause and effect to come (and the interconnected whole).

When we focus on the people exposed to toxins like McDonald's, cigarette smoke, or viruses that don't get sick as our baseline, we can establish a NEW normal. This new normal is establishing the common denominators that are present in those experiencing peace and wellness incorporating their entire focus.

Illness is caused internally. Healing is an internal process. We have been brainwashed for thousands of years to believe that people better than us with special powers of knowledge heal us or that magic pills heal us. The science proves otherwise. Treatments do not heal you. Healing comes from within. Fasting is an internal process that, if it gets confused with a treatment, may become external and fleeting.

GHOSTS, ANGELS, HEALING HANDS
AND GOD

The fact that most Americans believe in angels and ghosts is intriguing and fascinating. Eighty percent believe in angels, 50 percent believe in ghosts and about 70 percent believe you can be healed physically or supernaturally by God. Ninety percent of us believe in God. Then we have over 70 percent of the population on prescription drugs and 10 percent on recreational drugs. I have asked the question: *"Is taking drugs making the assumption that you are smarter than God?"* If we believe in the spirit and believe that the spirit heals then when belief is tested we turn to drugs or the external… We have a dilemma. Do we only believe in God when it's comfortable and/or it suits us?

Is our belief of the spirit magical thinking or is the belief based upon the principles of miracles? Is your belief in the spirit misguided or misdirected? That is to say that if we believe in the spirit as a form of magical thinking then we are separate from it. What I propose is a correct belief in the spirit: If you have a connection with your God, your Grand Purpose, and most importantly yourself—one interconnected whole—only then can you believe in these spirits and use them as miracles versus magic.

When someone goes to the person with "healing hands" and they walk again or have a profound change in their physical symptom, it will only last and be a miracle if the persons giving and receiving are on an equal playing field. If the receiver thinks of this person as a god, or "healer," or external, the results will be temporary and fleeting.

Is it useless to believe in a God that you cannot connect to when you need it? If your ladder is up against the wrong wall your belief may be built on sand. If your belief in the spirit (God, angel, healing hand) is outside you, it may be a superstition.

SECTION 2
ORDER AND MOTION

"Energy and Matter are two aspects of the same thing."
GustoveLeBon

Everything happens for a reason. What is the purpose of volcanoes? What is the purpose of an economic recession? What is the purpose of the common cold? Forest fires? Understanding the constructive aspects versus the destructive aspects is essential.

We tend to accept the constructive aspect of the volcano spreading alkaline ash minerals and cooling or heating the earth, yet condemn the destructive aspect of the volcano burning homes. Being selective in nature or natural consequences makes it impossible to heal. By deciding that a condition is a random mistake, genetic or bad luck, you miss the chance or possibility to heal. Does the forest fire "heal" the forest? Does it intend to bring the forest to a state of wholeness? Absolutely! There are not any cures in nature. In talking with my wise financial friend on the purpose of the cycles of recessions, he explains it is necessary for the economy; it is akin to a leaning-down process that makes the whole system more competitive and stronger.

Without getting emotional or personal, there is a purpose in all things that happen. If you don't know the purpose of the event or condition it does not mean that there is not a purpose, or that the event or condition was random, due to luck, or due to chance. Our universe, physics, and lives are based upon order and motion. Some may call it God's will or Karma or Cause and Effect. (In no way is this book claiming cause and effect is punishment for bad acts... stay tuned).

For the 10 percent of those who don't believe in a God, many through deductive reason believe in a God indirectly by accepting that there is order and motion and it is governed by a connective force that is proven in science. The Course In Health Workbook offers some cause and effect connections to our body parts. Clinically I have seen the connection between body parts and emotional links. Even mainstream medicine has studied and verified body parts with emotional connection. If the doctor or medical school has not found the connection or purpose of the condition as it relates to the condition doesn't mean there is not one. Just because it was not yet proven that the earth was not the center of the universe, doesn't mean it was.

You are truly empowered when you believe that everything happens for a reason versus luck, chance, and genetics. The ability to change and heal lies within you. Your focus must be something **Grand**.

In practice, I have found a large disconnect between patients and nature. I suggest the disconnect stems from not recognizing order and motion. Fifteen years ago I started teaching cooking classes and teaching patients about gardening. In teaching the quality of our health is directly related to the quality of our soil required lots of patience. When we look to build our home we want to use the best materials for obvious reasons. The same should apply to the quality of food we eat yet many overlook the quality ingredients for cheap alternatives. This is not a sales pitch for organic food. It is to point out that the reason most conventional food would be eaten by bugs if it was not sprayed by chemicals is to help us create order in health. I will explain why later.

ILLNESS IS A GOAL -
ORIENTED, BIOLOGICAL PROCESS

All illness is goal-oriented and purposeful in nature. There is no mistake about its process. The mainstream and natural medical approach believes the germ theory supersedes this by claiming bugs cause illness. There is no mistake that we have billions of bacteria and microbes in our eyes, throat, skin, and in our intestines. Like all body parts, the bacteria and microorganisms have a purpose. We have been taught that some bacteria are good and some are bad. I propose that all of these bugs are purposeful and useful. More specifically we are told that streptococcus is bad and lactobacillus is good. Why is it then that all healthy humans have E-coli or streptococcus in their gut and strep in their throat?

Your body is born bacteria free, and then by age three, your body has more microbes than human cells. Scientists have discovered that 99 percent of your genetic information comes from your bacteria/ microbe, not from your parents or family. At the same time, your microbes get passed down from your parents and your environment. The bacteria in our eyes, throat, gut, etc. are crucial for life. Without it, we would die. The bacteria are there for a reason. Let's explore why bugs are everywhere.

We acquire microbes starting at birth, traveling through the birth canal, then, through the foods we consume starting with breastmilk and skin contact with parents.

The confusion is created by the paradox we have with our thoughts on bacteria. We have been taught that bacteria can kill us, or make us very sick: from pneumonia or tuberculosis to urinary tract infection to strep throat to pink eye.

We are also exposed to fungus, parasites, and viruses with each breath we breathe. The association we have with all these microbes is negative as taught by our medical system. We have been taught that these microbes are bad and to stay healthy is to stay away from microbes. The fact is that microbes are a part of the cleaning system that helps digest and eliminate dead or sick cells. Microbes don't flourish when more food (dead cells) exists in the body. Flies don't create garbage as much as bacteria create dead cells or sick cells.

The amazing connection between the gut and the microbes of our mental state (cognition and self-control) has been researched and proven. I had one patient who, if she didn't take her enteric-coated probiotics would by her own account act out of control emotionally (This example could be because of several reasons). These bugs are so incredibly purposeful in creating homeostasis and health.

COLD TO CANCER
THERE IS A GRAND PURPOSE IN ALL ILLNESS

The Germ Theory changed modern medicine in the mid-1900s when Louis Pasteur stated, *"Kill the bug cure the disease."* With this change in modern medicine, we have stagnated healing in many ways. Why is it that some bugs foster health, while others make you sick? Why do some bacteria do both? How does the quote "the bug is of little significance if the environment is in order" upset or contradict Pasteur's original stance?

Consider Helicobacter pylori, the bacteria implicated in causing stomach ulcers. These bacteria were once found in the majority of the population, but their prevalence has steadily been decreasing and today only about half of the world's population has it. Most people with bacteria do not have ulcers or symptoms, but a small number develop painful ulcers in an acidic part of the digestive tract (a finding that earned a Nobel Prize in Medicine in 2005).

Helicobacter infections are treatable with antibiotics, but there's a twist: Blaser and colleagues have found that the absence of Helicobacter appears to be associated with diseases of the esophagus, such as reflux esophagitis and certain cancers of the esophagus. In other words, Helicobacter may be bad for our stomach, but good for our throat. Though not all scientists agree, "there's a big body of evidence that Helicobacter has both biological costs and biological benefits, Blasertold LiveScience. Tiny & Nasty: Images of Things That Make Us Sick.

Of the 1000 species of bacteria on our skin, we wouldn't want to live without them. They are beneficial to our health. The purpose of these billions of bugs is to act as a defense shield from unwanted things getting into our bodies; they are crucial to our immune system. If you don't believe this, bleach your skin daily to kill off these bacteria and see what happens to your health. It would become life-threatening. If you have ever seen someone in a burn unit you will quickly realize how the skin and bacteria protecting our bodies are crucial to life.

Most people are aware that there are healthy and unhealthy bacteria in our mouth. The normal flora/bacteria protect your teeth and gums from illness or decay. Unhealthy bacteria do the opposite and cause oral illness and can also cause heart problems. The unhealthy bacteria are only present when an illness is present. It is the illness that allows the bugs to grow and infiltrate, while at the same time the bugs are present before illness as a part of the immune system.

The same bacteria principles apply to all our body systems. We need bacteria.

Normal Flora of the Respiratory Tract

Normal Flora of the Urinary tract

Normal Flora of the Eye

Normal Flora of the Mouth

Normal Flora of the Gut

Think about the money spent on antibiotics and the money spent on probiotics. One kills bacteria and one supports and feeds bacteria. Why did our Creator put bacteria all over our body? Why do some bacteria and bugs make us sick? Hang tight the answer is coming.

An interesting point is that most, if not all cancers are tied to virus, bacteria or fungus. These are some of the cancers linked to out-of-balanced viruses:

Cervical & Prostate Cancer = HPV

Lung cancer = Chlamydia

Stomach Cancer = Helicobacter Pylori

Colorectal Cancer = streptococcus

Salmonella = Gallbladder

Liver Cancer = Hepatitis Virus

Non-Hodgkin's lymphoma = Epstein-Barr Virus

Skin Cancer = Granuloma type Virus

Bladder Cancer = Schistosomiasis

Hairy-cell leukemia = Retrovirus (HTLV-2)

Brain Cancer = Simian Virus 40

Leukemia = Fungus

With cancer and the bug connection being scientifically accepted, we should be focusing more attention on the simple beginnings of the virus or bug and addressing these differently—not the end result of the virus causing a gene to mutate.

The connection between bug and cancer is real, yet short-sighted when cause and effect are considered. It is simply missing the forest for the trees. We need to step back and observe the bigger picture of cause and effect. At some point, our thoughts will shift and we will accept the science that proves the virus and bacteria cannot be the cause of illness because they are a part of the body's natural environment. For example, a healthy person has staph bacteria on their skin and nose. It only grows uncontrollably when the immune system is off. So how can we say it is the cause?

What is the difference between a cold and cancer? A cold is a virus that takes hold in the host—you—when you are run down. The virus has a purpose: to slow you down by causing lethargy and fever. The high temperature slows down your mental processes allowing you to think and process why you are run down. If you respect that your body is speaking to you, you would then rest, drink plenty of water and address the causative factors. If you treat the virus as a mistake or bad luck and try to override the symptoms with drugs, this stimulates the possibility of the virus hanging around and progressing.

WHAT IS THE PURPOSE OF GETTING SICK?

There is no doubt that the virus and bacteria have an amazing purpose in our lives. When a virus goes unchecked in a weakened or stressed immune system, it will have the opportunity to alter genes and progress to mutate cells and grow. Your cold or your cancer is purposeful and intended to restore you back to health. The purpose of getting a cold is often overlooked or poorly understood. We get a cold because we are run down; the cold helps us slow down and re-center. There is always a lesson you can learn about this biological process. Pain management obscures and delays an illness' goal of restoring us back to health. Pain management stops the process of listening to yourself. We need to take a step back and ask what the pain is attempting to communicate with us, or what is the purpose of pain. The pain and inflammation with a sprained ankle are helpful to deter you from further injuring the ankle. It gives you feedback that is very helpful. If you could somehow make the pain go away and continue on the ankle the results would be damaging, turning from a sprain to a break.

Today many people are quick to cover up the pain. The concern is that the pain can't be tolerated, or shouldn't be tolerated, and that the pain is a mistake of nature. We then interfere with the goal the pain signals to us. Those who embrace pain are questioned as being martyrs or unstable. Most addictions are centered on avoiding pain. The important question is: "What is the purpose of pain?" This can simply be answered by seeing pain as a warning that something we are doing is "off the mark."

The typical response is to blame or feel sorry for yourself after a diagnosis of cancer. The usual dialogue would go something like *poor me or why me? Am I being punished? Am I just unlucky? It must be genetics. I better support the research foundations so they can come up with a cure before this thing gets me. Maybe there are some magic herbs that will cure this thing. I've got to beat it.* This dialogue focuses on the external cause and external cure. The complete paradigm dialogue would ideally ask the questions: What is the purpose of this? What is my body trying to tell me? How or why did I bring this into my life? (No blame). What areas of my life were not in order which may have contributed to this condition? What can I learn from this? The second dialogue is so much more empowering because of the understanding of where and why this condition manifested. This understanding of where and why we create these conditions and how to learn from them is the main purpose of this book. The other distinct difference is that the second approach offers no blame or guilt.

Many people have not been diagnosed with cancer and may not relate to the above dialogue. Let us look at a dialogue which most people can relate to: the common cold. The incomplete paradigm dialogue goes something like this: That darn flu bug is going around again. One of my coworkers had it, and I caught it. My son got his ear infection from another child at daycare. I guess I will need some cold medicine, or herbs or antibiotics. Cause "external" - Cure "external".

The complete paradigm dialogue would go like this: Bugs are naturally occurring in my system. These bugs go rogue when my balance is off. How or why did I allow my body to be a proper breeding ground for this bug? What areas of my life need to be altered or addressed? Why am I not getting enough sleep? Why am I so hurried, worried, etc.? What is this condition trying to tell me? Is it telling me to slow down? Is it telling me to look at my job dissatisfaction? Thank God that my body has allowed the virus or bacteria in to help digest my sick or dead cells. What I need to do is slow down and fill up my fuel tank. Cause "internal" - Cure "internal".

Does the mosquito create the swamp or the swamp attract the mosquito? I have posed this question to many patients with many being perplexed by the answer. We have been conditioned to believe that we catch the bug from other people or contact with objects based upon the theory of Louis Pasteur: "Kill the bug cure the disease." However, the science of bacteria supports that "the bug is of little significance if the internal environment is in order." When you allow your internal environment to get off balance, it provides the proper breeding ground for the bug. An analogy is that of a swimming pool, hot tub or fish tank. If you were to put all the right chemicals in a pool—to make it pH balanced—what are the chances of green algae or bugs growing in it? The chances are slim. Now, what if we neglected the pool for a year? The chemistry of the pool would shift, thus providing a proper breeding ground for bugs and algae. This same principle holds true with your body; when we neglect our bodies over time, we drift to unhealthy habits and choices, which shifts the body chemistry away from normal. The bug now has a proper breeding ground and has an open invitation from your body. The question that should be asked: Does the mosquito create the swamp or does the swamp attract the mosquito? The answer should be obvious, yet many have a difficult time embracing. They have been brainwashed that the swamp creates the mosquito by the medical system model. Or that flies create garbage. The earth is the center of the universe because the church or authorities state so...

The fact is these viruses are asexual, they are not alive, and they require a sick cell to reproduce. Bacteria and fungus are different in that they can reproduce. Bacteria and fungus can reproduce asexually and spread; this supports the sanitation efforts that have changed healthcare by simply understanding hygiene. It must be stressed that all of these microbes are opportunistic and require a sick person to thrive. Furthermore, having these microbes enter into the bloodstream through blood transfusion, contaminated needles or other unnatural means is not advised. Stay away from contaminated needles, or anything that would have direct access to your bloodstream. (Interesting to point out the biblical connections to menstruation and intercourse and blood transfusion)

For the unscientific denialist that would make false claims about this book's stance. I agree that unnatural bacteria exposure to our system will cause illness. I do not blame the bacteria; I ask why and how did the bacteria have access to a place protected by our Creator, along with the same questions as to why healthy people exposed in these unnatural ways don't get sick. Going off on a little tangent may help here. When the US dropped an atomic bomb on Japan the radiation exposure was real and damaging. The question seldom asked is how and why so many people exposed to the same levels of radiation did not get sick while others developed illness. The radiation being akin to the bacteria, unnatural exposure is not advised. Radiation is a natural aspect of our universe and like bacteria it serves a purpose. When a healthy person is exposed to natural or unnatural levels of radiation through the sun or living in the mountains—or unnatural ways like flying in airplanes, X-ray exposure, or atomic bombs—our body has a way of dealing with the oxidative stress/free radicals: our body's natural defense called antioxidants. This is similar to the way a healthy person deals with bacteria or fungal exposure, be it natural or unnatural.

This is why healthy people don't get sick just because someone else in the room has a cold. If the bug could talk he would say: "It is too hard to duplicate myself in this person. I will pick a weaker person." Many will want to resist and insist that there are certain conditions that are beyond control, like catching lice for example. Again, we ask the question: Why doesn't everyone who is exposed to lice catch lice? The environment of a child/person who gets lice must be conducive to the lice. Clinically, I have seen an essential fatty acid deficiency in children who get lice and are slow to get rid of them. The same is true for those who get bitten frequently by mosquitoes. Usually, I find that the individual is lacking certain B-complex vitamins. At this point, we need to dig more deeply and ask: Why are these particular people lacking in these particular vitamins or nutrients?

The common cold is a virus and your body chemistry can turn from balanced to unbalanced (swamp). A hot tub can turn from a clean bathing tub to a swamp tub. How you go from clean to the swamp is by ignoring the tub and not cleaning it. The PH balance and makeup of a bug changes—turning it into swamp water.

In humans, this happens when we lack sleep, water, nutrients, have too much caffeine, job stress, family stress, financial stress, and/ or relationship stress. It is important to stress that body chemistry or balance is without a doubt affected by all these factors. Analyzing all these factors may seem daunting. With the tools and exercises given in the workbook, these stresses become better understood The Course In Health Workbook.

By changing your chemistry from homeostasis to swamp and then being exposed to the virus, the virus decides that our swamp is a hospitable place to hang out. If the same virus passes by the healthy, balanced person, it decides that it could not survive in that environment. It is why you don't get sick every time you are in contact with a virus. In a little more scientific explanation, if the microbe has no dead or sick cells to thrive on it doesn't take residence.

Physiologically, the common cold is caused internally. What is the purpose of your body chemistry turning from homeostasis to a swamp? This is the crucial basis for understanding how illness is a goal-oriented, biological process. The purpose of a shift of homeostasis is to attract the virus. Yes, your body wants the virus and essentially craves to get sick in this scenario. The reason is that the virus will aid in cleaning up dead cells, and then give you a fever. The fever will slow down body processes; the high temperature slows thinking, making you tired so you sleep. When this process slows down your thinking, you are then able to reassess your behavior, thoughts and dietary choices which changed your body chemistry to a swamp. The fever increases your body temperature that will kill off the bug naturally and you will also naturally crave water, rest and nutritious foods. These restorative healthy combinations move or shift your body chemistry back to homeostasis. The purpose of the virus is beneficial in teaching us what we are doing is "off" and what makes our chemistry shift to the swamp. The reality is that you would not be moved to change your behavior/choices if you didn't attract the virus; therefore we conclude that the virus has a purpose.

There is a direct connection between soil health and the plants produced by them. The same connection applies to your health. I have studied soils and farming practices for the purpose of my medical practice. I used to drive several hours to meet with Dr. Robertson in

Higginsville Missouri as a mentor. One story that has stuck with me in my practice for 20 plus years is when he explained that when alfalfa was grown naturally with all the correct nutrients, bugs would stay away from it. He taught me extensively about the refractive index and sugar amount in the plant/alfalfa. When the alfalfa was healthy and had a refractive index above 20, the bugs would attempt to eat it and you could sometimes see the bug explode in the sunlight. The bugs ultimately learned not to eat that crop. He further explained how he watched the alfalfa crop adjacent to the healthy one get eaten by the bugs due to being a weak plant. A basic question not asked is why some crops get eaten and others don't. In natural selection, the healthy crop is strong and survives. The healthy crop has more nutrients and is better suited to sustain life by those consuming it. On the other hand, nature is doing us a favor by having bugs eat the weak inferior crop, taking them out of the food chain.

Another lesson from Dr. Robertson that was impressive was a study that he personally conducted in his town. He took hair samples and blood samples from many people on the same street with similar exposures. The hair samples looked at lead levels and the blood samples looked at calcium levels. What he found was that those who had high lead levels had below-normal levels of calcium in their body. Both lead and calcium are minerals. He explained that when people had healthy levels of calcium in their tissues, the body picked the calcium over the lead and eliminated the lead. When the body was deficient in calcium the body picked up (needed) the lead as a desperate second choice. We all know that lead exposure is not good, but the true lesson is that when you are healthy and balanced, exposure to lead is not that much of a concern.

The next question I had was why some people have low calcium levels, of which Dr. Robertson gave me much insight.

Your body innately knows how to repair itself. The same logic can be applied to cancer or any other condition. Perhaps you are beginning to see that there is always one more question you can ask when you are tempted to stop at the external explanation.

Your body innately knows how to repair itself – the increase in body temperature (fever) will hamper the growth of the virus – viruses don't live in a fever state for long. This allows the white blood cells to capture and remove the offending virus.

It is interesting to reflect on my own focus when I get the flu. My initial knee-jerk is to blame or find someone or something to blame; I try to recall what I ate and who I was in contact with. I have learned a new focus that I share in the workbook.

Crossroads: If you don't believe that there is a purpose in getting sick you will be unable to believe in healing. The germ theory falsely affirms the belief that there is no purpose in getting sick. The facts support otherwise.

THE PURPOSE OF PAIN...

...is to embrace and change

P U R P O S E
A C C E P T I N G
I N T E R N A L
N E E D S

Illness and pain are purposeful. We automatically assume that illness is bad or evil, when in fact the opposite is true. Illness is the doorway through which we may pass to healing. Illness is a goal-oriented, biological process. Understanding the two components may be helpful to you. Pain and pleasure are connected neurologically. Pain meds actually inhibit our sense of pleasure. Without pain, we cannot experience pleasure.

One of the biggest blocks to embracing pain is the idea that pain is punishment. If you have this sad belief in pain and punishment you are likely to mask the pain or seek blame.

First, there is a constructive aspect: that of bringing you back to normal (homeostasis). This can be observed for instance when your body invites a virus or bacteria. The body's response is to increase the core temperature with a fever to eliminate the bug. So the real purpose of the bug is to encourage you to slow down, get more rest, take a look at your relationships, your diet, etc. The purpose of the fever is to restore normal body chemistry.

If symptoms are suppressed the constructive part leads to the second part of the illness process which is destructive. The purpose here is to recycle or bring back to the soil. Have you ever seen a tree fallen in the woods and over time decompose and begin to return to the soil? Many of the patients I deal with are in the first stage of the process, the constructive aspect. Their body is seeking to repair and rebuild. If the patient continually insists on covering up the symptoms, whether with drugs, herbs, surgery or a myriad of other distractions, then the progression of illness takes over. The second stage of the illness process involves cancer, diabetes, autoimmune conditions, obesity, etc. To state the morbid reality: the second phase of the illness process is closer to death or *back to the soil*. It would be safe to say that both aspects are purposeful and meaningful. The second phase is not doom and gloom for certain. Through principles in healing, you can often reverse and keep latent the second phase.

Your immediate question might be "How is cancer purposeful?" All symptoms—pain, discomfort, etc.—are your body's way of communicating with you, telling you that what you are doing is not serving you. This may be clear and easy when manifesting the common cold. A person with clarity will say that the reason I manifested this cold was due to my daily choices. Not getting enough sleep, eating too much McDonald's, being stressed at work, etc. When this happens, your body chemistry will shift away from normal. Your body is in constant flux and will do everything it can to maintain homeostasis (balance). Your body will also give you clues. The first clue may present as fatigue. Most people will ignore this first attempt at communication and use stimulants to combat this fatigue. This will further move body chemistry away from balance.

In looking at the condition called 'cancer' the purpose is still present. A physics-based approach called 'atavistic' shows that cancer is a 'safe mode' for stressed cells. It claims that cancer which has been around for millions of years is a re-expression of a "preprogrammed" trait that was lying dormant. The analogy used is like our computers running in safe-mode when exposed to a serious threat. The problem or threat is uncovering the addiction or action (emotional condition) that has caused the stressed-out cells to need to be placed in safe-mode and then taking away the insult (carcinogen) in order to heal. Even if the atavistic model is not correct there is an explanation for the purpose and function of the etiology.

Finding the meaning and purpose of suffering and pain can be difficult at times. If we don't know the cause, it doesn't mean the cause doesn't exist. If the cause is coming from an emotional place and our questions are not framed to include the emotional cause, the purpose will elude us. "Ask and you shall receive" is so powerful—if and only if—you ask. To "find the gold in the womb" is the goal. Without fail, there is a lesson or reason (meaning) for suffering. It is our personal challenge to find out what has to be learned about our situation. How do we need to change our lives, our actions, our beliefs, our old hurts? Without fail, I have consistently seen the emotional link to any or all physical conditions. The challenge or difficulty is that many people are either not ready or not open to this connection.

When there is a realization that our illness is truly a result of our emotions, feelings, or internal conflict... we have made a huge step. Truly believing is different than entertaining the possibility that it might be partially due to my emotions and continuing to hold onto the incomplete paradigm.

The investment (or need) we have in our condition serves the ego to defend the condition and look for external remedies. The extent of the investment or comfort of the condition is the extent of disabling the healing. For example, I have had a glimpse of this condition that I have experienced since childhood start to clear up. For a slight moment, I felt lost without it. It was part of me. I believe everybody does this. Connecting with the comfort of the condition is difficult to recognize because we block this as a possibility. It takes swallowing my pride to admit such thing. I am almost embarrassed to admit it. However, it taught me the importance of focusing my attention on my thoughts and happiness. This concept is abstract and difficult to articulate. Others call this "loving your condition." In the workbook, we discuss the secondary gains associated with illness and conflict. It is the secondary gain that gets missed with why we get sick.

Let's go back to the paradox of not having to have a natural diet or exercising regularly to live a strong healthy life. In identifying the common traits of those who enjoy health without exercise, for example, the common denominator is a Grand Purpose and a level of congruence and peace in their lives. I have spent a great deal of my practice and research on those who don't get sick despite ignoring timeless health principles. Take the person who smoked a pack or two for 50 years, and lived well into their 90s or the 90-year-old who never exercised. They are not the poster children for Whole Foods market or Gold's Gym. Many people will take these testimonies and rationalize their behavior around them. I would be all for this if the person taking the testimonial of the smoker or non-exerciser applied the whole picture of the testimonial to include their emotional makeup.

We must take the leap to addictions to fully understand the paradox. The person who smoked all his life and did not develop illness did so because the congruence, balance, and purpose in his life as a whole offset the negative effects of smoking, and possibly the smoking was an aide to his life. Most likely this person was not addicted to the smoking in a way that undermined his foundation of purpose or health. More so, the person not addicted can and will walk away from the substance or behavior with little or no resistance if their purpose is challenged by it. In this stance it answers how and why many can drink or smoke their entire life and not have illness; the same applies to coffee, food, work, etc.

Addiction is defined in two ways: 1) A strong need to engage in an activity, substance, or thing that is rewarding YET harmful; 2) A strong need to engage in an activity, substance, or thing that is rewarding.

The gray area is when the strong need is driven by a lack of self-control versus purpose and drive. Almost everything in life has the ability to be habit-forming or addictive. The behavior or addiction is relative to one's self-control. Exercise, for example, is also habit forming; once you get the tight, flexible, strong body, you become addicted to the benefits and it is difficult to stop exercising. Your career or job is the same. Once you receive positive feedback and reward (financial and emotional) you become addicted to working and it is difficult to stop receiving the financial and emotional rewards of this behavior. There is no question that people who exercise or work can stop if required to do so.

Those who consume prescription drugs, alcohol, street drugs, or gamble have all received positive secondary gains, feedback or benefits.

The secondary gain of drugs or alcohol may be "perceived joy." I had one person tell me that his secondary gain of drinking alcohol was he became funnier, sold more and made more money. For all those addicted they weigh the secondary gain above the primary cost of the addiction.

These secondary gains cause an addiction. There is also no question that stopping these addictions is doable. One of the keys to understanding that the person is bigger than the addiction is when purpose and self-control are addressed and the need for these things is outweighed by the costs.

For those addicted to being financially messed up or those who are addicted to dysfunctional relationships, they must stop and question all of it and address how they are connected and what secondary gain they receive from the addiction. There is always a secondary gain otherwise there would be no addiction.

The medical system now calls gambling, drugs, alcohol, and sex addictions a "disease." I believe that it is a slippery slope to do so. Much of calling these addictions "disease" is purely for financial reasons, insurance billing and to prescribe meds. Without a "disease," insurance companies can't pay for treatment. You can't prescribe drugs or treatment for something that is not a disease, according to the system. This is a slippery slope... If the medical system does not stop here, does it label anyone in debt with a "financial disease"? Does the pattern continue in labeling those committing crimes as having a "disease"?

This is justified by the fact that the need to spend more than you make is a pattern that gives short-term gratification or pleasure for those who do so. Next, they would have to label those in unfulfilling relationships to be addicted. People who drink soda or coffee daily would also require a diagnosis and label of disease/addiction.

When someone starts to drink or smoke or use drugs, they are not consciously saying to themselves *I have stress that I don't want to address, I will drink until the alcohol becomes a problem in my life, threatens my physical health, my marriage, my job or my freedom. When this happens I will hit rock bottom and address the issues that led me to drink.* We can generalize that the process of drinking (or drugs) goes something like this: overwhelming stress or low self-esteem, combined with poor coping skills... The alcohol helps numb the pain and discomfort of the stress. The alcohol's short-term positive effect of suppressing symptoms makes it easy to ignore the deep problems or issues and focus on the benefit of alcohol's pleasure. Because illness is a goal-orientated, biological process and its focus is to return us to health, we ultimately and subconsciously want to resolve and heal. The common denominator in healing the addiction is a realization that the alcohol was a tool to bring them to their conflict. The alcohol was used in the process of healing. Even though alcohol has a destructive component evident in the harm it does to the physical body, along with other negative-destructive components like interfering with your job, or your ability to function, the destructive component has a purpose. The constructive aspect of alcohol is that it makes you feel good temporarily, it is a stress reliever, and it inhibits your emotions, etc. The most constructive aspect of alcohol is that it will allow you to hit rock bottom if you require so – in order to change. You can change the alcohol analogy to smoking, gambling, prescription drugs, food, etc. Just as money is not evil—drugs or alcohol, shopping or gambling—are not as well. They are often associated with bringing people to their crossroads.

The next big leap is to see the similarity between all illnesses: Heart illness, cancer, diabetes, Alzheimer's, etc. They are no different from the process of addiction to drugs, alcohol or smoking. And yes these illnesses are a form of addiction. To create heart illness you must be committed to or addicted to certain behaviors, foods, thoughts, feelings, and projections; you must be committed to lifestyle choices that help support the physiology of heart illness and most importantly… your refusal to CHANGE.

With the purpose of illness to bring us back to health and/or to become whole, where does the "cure" fit in? Does making a symptom go away bring us any closer to healing or becoming whole? Or further away? The correct interpretation of the preceding is that illness is purposeful and connected to principles in nature. It is not a punishment tied to guilt or evil. It is a gentle way in which the vice brings us back to connection. My clinical experience is that most people are looking for cures/magic in the process of illness. The shame and guilt of getting an illness make us all uncomfortable so we just want to make it go away.

In summary, pain either gently or loudly tells us that something we are doing is opposite to our Grand Purpose.

DO NOT LABEL YOUR CONDITIONS

One of the greatest disservices the medical profession (natural included) does is label conditions by giving them names. When we label a condition we automatically associate the label of "disease" as being something external (outside of ourselves), and beyond our control. When this happens, a subconscious blocking of internal control naturally and predictably happens. It becomes mystical and more real with the naming of the illness and giving the disease a name.

The difference is real. Think about the difference between your natural or medical doctor telling you that you are depressed versus you are depressing. Think of the difference in your thinking between being told you have some inflammation or irritation in your gut versus being told you have ulcerative colitis or Crohn's disease or cancer. With the latter, most think about genetics and then start thinking about what medication or treatment is necessary. When you ask the doctor what causes ulcerative colitis, they respond "we don't know" or "it's genetic." When addressing the condition as inflammation or irritation we are more likely to be empowered. What is irritating my gut? What can I do to help reduce inflammation? You also look at the condition as temporary versus permanent. You may ask why ulcerative colitis or Crohn's disease doesn't prevail in many parts of the world.

The naming of symptoms into a "disease" shifts the illness from internal to external and from more temporary to more permanent. In the workbook, this is a key exercise. Compare saying "I have a disease called depression" versus saying "at times I feel and act low" or even better "I am depressing." Clearly for the person seeking to heal they will opt for the temporary and internal approach to owning it.

The same applies to mental disorders and addictions. When someone is labeled 'bipolar' versus 'stressed out', the same process as above plays out. The labeled condition becomes pessimistic thus seen as permanent requiring medication or treatment. Mental disorders are just groups of symptoms that lead to a diagnosis of a "disease."

A group of doctors in 1952 created these mental diseases. The National Institute of Mental Health claims that the DSM (Diagnostic and Statistical Manual of Mental Disorders) represents an irrational and subjective system and no longer supports projects that rely entirely on DSM criteria. The creation of conditions to satisfy insurance companies and create billable claims from drugs to therapy needs to be questioned and dismantled. Some of the highly controversial diagnoses include Gender Identity Disorder, Sex addiction, **Homosexuality, Childhood bipolar disorder, and Adult ADHD. (**Homosexuality was removed as a disease in the 1970s)

By embracing the complete paradigm in this book, people get lasting results, without the psychological damage and shame as having a thing called "disease." In the case of alcohol, we don't make the alcohol out to be some external thing that controls people. And yes, sex addicts, work addicts and shoppers all can continue to shop, work and enjoy sex. The concept of "diseases" is superstitious.

Beyond labeling mental disease, our medical system has created the most dangerous word associations of all time. When a person is told they have cancer, that event alone causes immense stress and possibly further harm. Where doctors can impart a placebo upon a patient, they also can provide a nocebo. The naming of conditions is disempowering for the patient and empowering for the doctor. The naming of patterns of symptoms is for the benefit of the doctor, not the patient. Arbitrarily giving a group of symptoms a name is seldom questioned. Who decided to make a group of symptoms of a disease and why have we accepted it? Except for insurance or to make the doctor feel superior, there is no purpose for naming conditions that aides the customer.

I believe the poor outcomes in cancer are primarily due to the crippling external focus on what cancer is and the name association some have accepted as truth. Overcoming the separation of the cancer being this thing outside of you that you must fight is nonsense. The other thought—that we must attack this external disease with force— is another unfounded focus. The concept of getting all cancer with surgery is one of the most unscientific claims made in medicine.

The bottom line is that healing becomes difficult or impossible when we label conditions. The empowering healing approach is to identify the illness from an internal vantage point. My body is inflamed; my homeostasis was off and wants to move back towards balance.

THE CAUSE OF ILLNESS...

...is the belief that healing is the enemy

Our current medical system places little to no emphasis on discovering the cause. The system is focused instead on symptoms, giving them a name, and then covering them up with drugs or surgery. Our natural doctors are doing the very same thing, with the exception of those who prescribe self-reflection, exercise, whole foods and those who address the addiction. The true cause of illness comes from one of two things:

By thinking about a condition. For example, after exposing yourself to someone with a cold, you say to yourself over and over again: "I am going to get sick." Or, perhaps your mother had breast cancer at the age of 44, and your thoughts are constantly replaying: "My mother had breast cancer, I probably will too."

The second and more common cause of illness is from our emotions: anger, resentment, guilt, worry, fear, and so forth. This leads us to choose the wrong behavior, such as picking the wrong doctor or choosing not to exercise. The cause is not hydrogenated oils, refined sugar, lack of exercise, chemotherapy or drugs. The reason is whatever emotion or conflict made us choose these behaviors.

Both involve a sense of separation from a higher purpose. A cure addresses symptoms and wants them suppressed by either natural or pharmacological processes. When is the last time your doctor has discussed the emotional root of your condition? Before you jump the gun and think this is just spiritual teaching, the preceding is based upon the science of cause and effect.

I would like to share a dialogue I had with a patient. He came to my office with some neck problems. He expressed to me that his former physician (chiropractor) had not satisfied him. He understood the different components of health, or thought he did (physical, structural and emotional) and that was why he came to me. I explained how the foods we eat play a profound effect on muscles, along with breathing, water consumption and emotions. During his second visit for an adjustment he asked me: "What causes this neck pain? My last chiropractor said the vertebra was out and it is interfering with the nerve." So I explained to him that muscles move bones, bones move muscles. In other words, muscle tension may cause the bone to go out of place. Muscle tension caused by stress...

Then he said, "So the real cause of my neck pain is muscle tension?" I then asked him what causes the muscle tension. He replied, "I get it. It's stress that causes the muscle tension, that causes the bone to go out of place, that irritates thenerve, that causes the pain." He almost had it. I asked him what is the difference between two people reacting completely different in a similar situation (I.e. the reason your neck muscles are stiff is because your boss yelled at you). How can it be then that your co-workers received the same tongue-lashing and shrugged it off with no resulting muscle tension? This patient ultimately reached the answer he was seeking simply by changing the question he was asking. (Research the cause of muscle tension on the internet.)

The medical research has begun to prove the above claim I make. There are mounds of studies showing the connection to emotions, personality types, and stress on all illness. No educated person would disagree that stress causes people to make poor personal choices, like smoking or drinking excessively, or eating poorly. No one can deny that these behaviors are linked to all illness conditions.

What if you subconsciously select or want and love your illness? I ease into this with the "what if" question. In those who genuinely heal they all have the same commonality in that they all agree that at some level they created, wanted, needed, or manifested their condition to get love (not saying guilt or blame).

Those ready to change and heal will focus on themselves and be willing to internalize and heal. They will ask "Do I love or create my illness?" Those with too much fear or guilt will start to challenge, and some even attack me on this teaching. If your knee-jerk reaction is to direct your attention to hypotheticals, exceptions or luck, chance or genetics—you will claim this is ridiculous. The child who got raped, the innocent person being hit by a drunk driver, the child who develops leukemia... are reason enough to support the old system. My response is always the same: How is that working for you? If you're not ready to shift from external to internal because the fear and guilt are too high, be gentle with yourself and be open.

47

THE TRIGGER

The trigger or root of all health problems is emotional. All illness—financial, relationship, and physical—is triggered by an addictive pattern/emotional trap. Many times the addictive trigger is not addressed or correlated to the condition, and therefore the correction or healing eludes; instead, we look for external cures like pills or treatments. Without exception, the addictive pattern is the biggest challenge to address and change. In searching for the cause, I have found that pointing out the possible addiction that is the trigger is often rejected by the patient. The patient pleads, "I don't think it is this or that," while choosing to believe or address other possible (external) causes.

I had a cancer patient who before her diagnosis ate well and exercised and was a hardworking mother who was loved and appreciated by her family and community. She came to me seeking advice on what approach she should take in taking on her cancer diagnosis. The one thing we addressed was her deep-seated resentment of putting others first and feeling controlled in her relationship. This self-sacrificing, addictive pattern was not easy to resolve because it had many benefits entangled in it. Many emotional patterns have positive secondary gains associated with them. A self-sacrificing person gets a lot of secondary benefit from giving—even though it is at their own expense and health. Once we identified the benefits she received from her cancer diagnosis (and self-sacrifice), she was able to address the pattern of addiction and reward. A similar analogy is an overachieving executive who gets many secondary financial gains by working hard, being unrelenting and meeting high standards. When the person is told that these unrelenting, overachieving standards are killing them by creating high blood pressure and a weakened immune system, the difficulty is the fear associated with giving up the high standards and secondary gains of being revered as successful. Going back to the cancer patient, it is sometimes too complicated for the self-sacrifice person to give up the addiction of self-sacrificing because the secondary gains of feeling needed are too challenging to overcome.

Cancer patients with an impending diagnosis are often more open to looking for the root cause and effect. When it comes to muscle tension (back pain), headaches or other pain we often are not compelled to address the addiction that causes discomfort. This can be compared to the high prevalence of people not discussing their retirement, and they have blinders on that it's not pressing.

Cause and Effect: When you go in for treatment—acupuncture, massage, chiropractic adjustment—or you take a pill, herb, or prescription and you get relief from your symptom—you are erroneously made to believe that the treatment fixed you. It is fair to connect the treatment to pain relief as a cause and effect. The problem is it is incredibly short-sighted. If you are heavy in debt and cannot pay rent and you go to a payday loan center and get a high-interest loan, your pain is gone! You can pay your rent. Is it a solution? Or, in reality, very short-sighted? We will discuss primary causes versus secondary causes.

What about this person? Or that person? Or children? My rule is to not talk in hypotheticals or about other people's conditions. Wanting to dissuade yourself from healing you look for ways to prove otherwise. If you look at your condition—and your condition only—with a level of honesty, you will be compelled to change.

The brainwashing that high blood pressure, obesity, inflamed joints or depression is luck, chance or genetics, allows us not to address the addiction. Almost always when I discuss what I believe is the addiction for the patient they disagree and want to focus on something else. *I think it's diet, doc… or I think I need this treatment.* The humble and wise come back and surrender to the emotional addiction and Wow! Does change happen.

Denialism: This book does not refute the connection between the illness and other proximate causes of illness. In frustration, some may misrepresent what this book says and claim it doesn't accept the hard science. Not true. This book respects the connection between virus and genes that are associated with many illnesses. This book claims that these are in NO way the proven causes of the illness. Someone close to you gets shot and hurt, the police only want to look at the bullet and gun. They are not looking for the person shooting the gun. The police officer determines the bullet and gun did the harm and you are crazy to question him to look any further because he found the cause! Then after years of watching this same pattern, you say the emperor is wearing no clothes. You say the officer is not addressing the cause of the gunshot. You say we need to address the shooter as the cause and they want to discredit you because you claim the bullet and gun are not the cause. Denialism is that the cause does not start with emotions.

THE COMPLETE PARADIGM
OR THE ACCURATE MAP

Many people have an aversion to hearing that prevention and taking responsibility for your health is the best insurance. Furthermore, making changes to one's lifestyle offers even more resistance. If you are excelling in these areas you don't have any issue with this information. It's the classic preaching to the choir. If you change the thinking from "taking responsibility" to "moving from an external focus to an internal focus" you get the same result and it's easier. For example, saving money for retirement is prevention and taking responsibility.

Health and happiness start by taking responsibility for how you feel—shifting the focus from external to internal. What does taking responsibility for one's health mean? The answer is in your choices, actions, thoughts, beliefs, and feelings. The claim that the majority of your health is a result of decisions is backed by many studies which have been reproduced to substantiate the connection. The problem is that our natural and modern medical doctors do not teach nor understand these connections.

Take into consideration that genetics and external treatments play a minimal role in your health (maybe 20-30%). Being responsible means being able to respond to the situation. Epigenetics has proven that the genes you have been dealt play a small role in your health.

The medical teaching that genetics and disease are a one-way street, or that your genetic makeup dictates your health has been proven to be false. The fact is that you do have control over your genes. Expression of your genetic makeup is determined by emotions, diet, lifestyle, and exercise. Put another way; you can be dealt a terrible hand in poker and still produce a winning hand. It is not the cards you are dealt, but how you handle them that counts. If your family has a history of heart disease, alcoholism, cancer or psychological problems it does not mean that they will manifest in you. The science behind Epigenetics proves solid.

When people shift responsibility, they are merely blaming. Scapegoats include but are not limited to genetics, bad luck, age, evil spirits, lack of money, etc. A study of the history of modern medicine shows us that the labels we have put on conditions and the mode of treatments have changed, but conditions are identical. A condition in the year 200 BC, 1600 AD and in the year 2019 all would have different labels and different modes of treatment, however, the condition is the same. For example, a headache in 200 BC could have been diagnosed as evil spirits or demons; today it is diagnosed into several categories of headaches. The bottom line is that the condition is the same, yet the name it is given changes. About 7000 years ago the medical doctors were fond of a technique they called skull trephining. This procedure consisted of drilling holes in the patient's skull to allow evil spirits to escape. Please note this was mainstream, accepted medicine at the time. Here you can see that the cause (evil spirits) was external, and the cure/treatment (drilling holes) was external. When this treatment became outmoded and deemed dangerous and ineffective, it was replaced by new treatments and interventions. Bloodletting is the practice of controlled bleeding to release demons from the body. Once again, the cause is external (demons), the treatment is external (bloodletting). Then antibiotics came to kill the bug and cure the patient. The cause (a bug) was external, and the cure (antibiotics), external. Then we have tonsillectomy: the cause, infection or virus (external), the cure (surgery), external. Today we see escalating numbers of patients turning to surgery to remove "diseased" organs. We see history repeating itself.

All these approaches follow the rules created by the same paradigm: that of external cause/cure (the rescue syndrome or the relinquishment of responsibility). Reviewing old medical approaches, we can see in hindsight that in time, all these procedures ceased. Accepting a diagnosis of evil spirits and then allowing a doctor to drill holes in the skull to remedy the issue? We scratch our heads in disbelief! I propose that the same disbelief will occur 40 years from today. In likelihood, our grandchildren will be astonished that we not only accepted diagnoses like cancer but added insult to injury by allowing doctors to give us chemotherapy (nerve gas) and lethal radiation. Medical research is proving that these treatments for cancer are ineffective and in most cases doing more harm than if patients did nothing at all, yet the procedures continue. The pattern is consistent: each treatment is proven ineffective and dangerous.

Most medical treatments (drugs, surgery, etc.) will cease because they will be proven harmful or substituted with a similar approach and a new sales pitch. To look at the history of medicine, we are given this obvious warning. Many if not all procedures and drugs of the past have been proven harmful. Unfortunately, they were quickly replaced with equally harmful and useless therapies. The vast majority of popular medications 20 years ago are no longer in circulation. Modern medicine would have you believe that we now have better drugs. The truth, however, is that the vast majority of older drugs have been proven ineffective, harmful, or both. For those who like to bring up exceptions and argue and say aspirin and other drugs have been around for years, yes, these drugs have been around and have also proven to be harmful. But big business and lack of action by the consumer encourage their existence. Aspirin use causes an astonishing 20 to 40 thousand deaths each year due to internal bleeding. This fact is ignored by the public and by the companies that are making billions off sales each year. Aspirin, Tylenol, and other painkillers are now proven to be deadly to liver and kidney function.

Over the last couple of years the amount of legal drugs advertised on television has skyrocketed. Listen to the commercials and the footnote side effects following. This drug may cause severe liver damage and this drug may cause heart problems, etc. It amazes me that a company can advertise a potentially fatal aspect of a drug, be open about it and realize that this commercial will help sales. This, I must say is the biggest slap in the face to the consumer. The old adage "buyer beware" doesn't apply. The drug pushers are giving you the information up front and most people selectively filter out and/or flat out ignore the facts given by the drug company. To the drug company's defense, they are giving people what they are asking for. If the drug is fatal in a small percentage of people taking it, then it is toxic in all cases. You may ask: "How is it toxic in ALL cases? Many people take it with no issues or side effect." If something is toxic, it is toxic. Our amazing, balanced body is built to neutralize and detox toxins. So even if you are healthy and strong and have the ability to mitigate the toxin, it is still toxic. The canary in the coal mine is the analogy that fits. In the olden days they would have a canary in the coal mine as a warning of dangerous gases being present. If the canary died the coal miners would leave promptly. The canary represents the one that the gas (drug) is toxic or fatal to— warning the others to leave before it is too late. The canary is the one person that displays toxic effect. RUN!

The downplaying of the warning stating that only in a small percentage is there a serious problem is unethical. Scientists know with certainty that 100 percent of the people will be faced with toxicity to varying degrees. Just picture a television advertisement for cocaine. If you are feeling down and out, you want to escape and feel powerful, take cocaine. The warning would be similar to the legal drug pushers: cocaine may cause heart problems in a small percentage of people.

Approximately 30 years ago the leading advertiser in the New England Journal of Medicine was the tobacco industry. Presently, it is pharmaceutical drug companies. The advertising for tobacco stopped for obvious reasons. Give it time and the present advertising will be deemed unethical. Today only two countries (the USA and New Zealand) have made it legal for drug companies to advertise and push drugs on television.

I estimate that 95 percent of the medical procedures and drugs used today will not survive the test of time and will be obsolete in 40-50 years for this very reason. I also believe only 20 percent of all natural and medical treatments and prescriptions are necessary and helpful. Remember tonsillectomies? The procedure comes in and out like a fad because the procedure has been deemed ineffective and dangerous. The American Academy of Otolaryngology-Head and Neck Surgery Foundation has published clinical practice guidelines, and these guidelines discourage this surgery. The medical research shows that this procedure is ineffective or only moderately effective.

Tonsils are a part of our immune system. They are one of the first lines of defense our body has against infection. Removing part of our immune system because it is inflamed makes little sense. The reasoning for removal is based on an inflammatory process that can't be controlled.

This practice has been around since 1000 BC. Interestingly it comes in and out of fashion.

The reason why the procedure is used is that doctors rarely focus on the cause of the tonsils being inflamed and rarely teach patients ways of minimizing stress and supporting the immune system. Doctors are often pressured by parents to do something. Removing the tonsils is what they know how to do and what they have been taught to do.

What is amazing is that very few doctors and patients challenge the common sense aspect of removing a portion of your immune system. The British Journal of General Practice conducts a MEDLINE search of the effectiveness of this procedure. The outcome reveals uncertainty and many adverse effects from this procedure. It also recommends caution in this procedure. Translation: Don't have the procedure done. So why are so many people undergoing unnecessary and dangerous procedures? I believe that these procedures allow for the people involved to avoid the real changes required to heal. These procedures enable parents to avoid change by blaming the condition on luck, chance or genetics.

Another example is arthroscopic knee surgery. Respected medical research has shown that patients who undergo a "sham surgery" (where the patient believes he has had surgery and didn't get the surgery) feel just as well as those who had the surgery. The conclusion: arthroscopic knee surgery is not helpful. To the disbelief of many, the doctors and patients continue to do the surgery. It is the definition of quackery at its best.

In revisiting history, we see how this external medical treatment comes in and out like a fad. We have another modern parallel: plastic tubes surgically implanted in an infant's ear. In fact, tubes have already been proven ineffective by medical science. Medical literature states that children who have no treatment fare better than those with intervention. Likewise, medical literature says that antibiotics for ear infections are ineffective and unproven. Why would doctors continue to use these two procedures in their practice? One can only guess at their reasons. Perhaps they are following the advice I saw on a bumper sticker: *"If it ain't broke, fix it 'til it is."* At a seminar I attended, I heard another joke from a doctor who put her ego aside long enough to tell this joke at least: *"Nothing is better for a headache than Tylenol. So do nothing."* The point here is that it seems the medical community feels it imperative to take action, even when they are aware that action is inappropriate. Are they being pushed towards this compulsion by their patients? I believe so. When a concerned parent brings their child to see a doctor, almost all parents expect the doctor to do something (external) for the child. Parents want their child's pain to go away, and parents are brainwashed into thinking that if you don't do something external you are off course. Watchful waiting and the educating of patients is seldom practiced in our medical system even though it has been proven highly effective. The majority of back pain and other musculoskeletal pain will resolve over time. When someone is seeing a chiropractor, physical therapist or whomever while the natural process of healing is happening, regardless of therapy, the results are mostly attributed to the treatment, not our body's ability to self-correct.

What about treatments—medical and natural—that have somewhat consistent and palliative support? What about acupuncture that helped the sinus infection or tennis elbow? Or the chiropractic adjustment that helped a headache? Or the surgery replacing a hip? Or the supplement or herb helping with a condition? Because of these consistent, inconsistent, and sometimes haphazard treatments, it adds tremendous confusion to health. One analogy that will help in some way is the effect of seeing a person win the lottery, or hearing the slot machine hit the jackpot. These examples are not accurate scientific accounts of gambling paying off. They are individual accounts that reinforce the addiction people have with wanting to get rich quick or take shortcuts. Yes, taking the supplement or drug is looking for a shortcut.

Because medicine pays off 10-20 percent of the time, does it mean it works? The same question for casinos: If the lottery paid off .0000001 percent of the time and the slot machine 20 percent of the time and the blackjack 40 percent of the time, does it mean that gambling is a viable way to make money? For the one that hits the jackpot, they may worship the casino or the lottery, but it is still not proven effective.

It is why I am so against testimonials for healthcare treatments. It is why testimonials in the lottery and gambling are destructive. They encourage people to become addicted to an illusion. The lottery ticket commercial is not any different from the drug commercial.

Gandhi once said, *"Every action that is directed by fear or by coercion of any kind ceases to be moral."* I see these scare tactics being employed by chiropractors, dentists, multi-level vitamin pushers, vaccine pushers, and medical doctors.

Our medical industry excels at emergency and trauma treatment. Unfortunately, this contribution has erroneously led people to attempt addressing their other health issues with dismal results. As of 1998, one-half of all North Americans will eventually experience heart disease. Over one-third will suffer from cancer. These are "illnesses of affluence" as are osteoporosis and diabetes. Eighty to ninety percent of these illnesses as well as other "degenerative illness" can be prevented and reversed if the real cause is addressed.

The single most important medical advance in history is modern sanitation systems such as sewer, toilets, garbage collection, and hand washing. These advances in sanitation occurred at approximately the same time as the inception of modern medicine, and unfortunately, their good results have been attributed to modern medicine model. Do not confuse this with the germ theory.

To understand the cause of a condition is to be able to "cure" the condition. Our medical system places virtually no emphasis on discovering the cause. You are led to believe that medicine looks for the cause. However, when the cause can't be fed a drug or vitamin or treatment it is because the cause is deeper: lifestyle or toxicity or emotional or addiction. The system is focused instead on symptoms; the system gives them a name, and then covers them up with drugs or surgery. Our natural doctors are doing the very same thing, except those who prescribe rest, exercise, posture, nutritious food, and clean water and air.

To illustrate the extent to which many of us are rooted in our current beliefs about health, we often ask people if they believe regular dental checkups are vital to the care of their teeth. Almost everybody responds with an emphatic "of course!" What if, for instance, your regular dental check-up reveals two cavities? After receiving your fillings, will you resume the lifestyle which led to those cavities, only to return in a few months to find more? For thousands of years, the Eskimo culture has been curiously free of dental cavities. Part of the reason for this is the simple fact that they eat ample amounts of essential fatty acids (whale blubber) and chew on hard substances (dried seal, caribou and whale meat). Their strong teeth are not the result of fluoride treatments or regular exams at the Igloos-R-Us Institute of Healthy Teeth. However, in the past 50 or so years, with the introduction of sodas, cookies and chips, white bread and other nutrient depleted foods, the Eskimos have experienced dental cavities at a rate higher than the rest of modern society. Similarly, we can look at the logic of having the 200 or so bones in our bodies checked on a regular basis by our chiropractor. After all, if we are dedicated to having 20 to 30 teeth examined on a regular basis, shouldn't we provide even more attention to the bones that protect our nervous system and allow us to move? We find our answer to this question by looking at Asians who for centuries included yoga exercises in their daily regime, allowing them to enjoy excellent musculoskeletal health. Their attitudes, diet and proper movement through yoga postures and movement, make regular spinal checks unnecessary. Proper movement and nutrition produce health. Let me reiterate the core of this book and what I hope to convey: Proper beliefs and thoughts are what lead us to these behaviors. It is clear that regular physical exams, spinal checks, and eye exams are for those who choose not to practice prevention. Which of the following mindsets do you find more satisfying? A clean bill of health from your doctor based on an array of diagnostic procedures (blood tests, x-rays, mammograms, etc.), or a clean bill of health from yourself, based on knowing with certainty that your lifestyle habits, relationships, thoughts, and beliefs are congruent with accessing the full potential or unlimited potential within you?

There is not a single physician in this world that knows more about your health than yourself. No one but you knows the specific life circumstances and millions of experiences that have shaped who you are today. You are your own best doctor. Having a doctor or coach help you access your health or heal is sometimes a help.

NO CONSPIRACY - JUST CORRUPTION

I do not believe there is any conspiracy within our healthcare system—corruption, yes. I don't think that the American Medical System is involved in a plot to undermine our health. I don't think the good people at big pharmaceuticals are trying to undermine your health. Just as I don't believe natural doctors and their associations are trying to undermine your health. However, each segment of our medical system relies on ignoring the cause to sell their product and service. Is it corruption or ignorance that allows for unnecessary and unproven treatments? Maybe just greed or justified compartmentalization…

"It is difficult to get a man to understand something when his salary depends on his not understanding it." Upton Sinclair

If natural and medical doctors started calling their work cover-up care, I would consider that "real" and sincere. Calling it healthcare is false advertising! Making claims of effectiveness without proof is also quackery. Not addressing the difference between cures and healing is reckless.

The snake oil salesman truly believes in the oil. I don't think that people who sell snake oil today or those of the past thought that they were crooks. Maybe just greed or justified compartmentalization allows them to continue. These salespeople become gullible and don't have the insight or self-awareness to determine otherwise. The same gullibility applies to the pharmaceutical rep. No difference! When the oil or the drug puts food on the table, it is difficult to question.

When the salesperson wants to sell the oil, they separate themselves from the customer and become the all-knowing, clairvoyant to get leverage on the customer. Changing healthcare requires putting the patient on equal footing with the doctor. Let's start this process of healing by calling you a "customer" of healthcare versus a "patient."

Patient (defined): *Bearing pains or trials calmly or without complaint; manifesting forbearance under provocation or strain.*

Let's start by calling ourselves a "customer" (or partners) for healthcare issues, counseling issues, legal issues, and financial counsel. No more "patient." You are customer paying for a service, seeking results. You may have a hard time believing that the medical system uses marketing strategies similar or greater than other industries. You would think that medicine and doctoring would succeed without advertising or marketing strategies. The fact is the money spent on the propaganda is alarming.

OUR INTERCONNECTED WHOLE

Finances and relationships have everything to do with our health. It is well-established that those businesses that adopt an internal framework of focus succeed; the same applies to relationships and finances. The many books that have shown these connections are well received. The same principles must be applied to health. The purpose of discussing relationships, finances and businesses are twofold: 1) To show those who successfully use the internal focus approach and 2) It is difficult—maybe not even possible—to separate finances and relationships with health, as they are all interrelated. Ask yourself if you can be healthy without being happy. Finances may cause stress that directly affects your health and vice versa. The same applies to your relationships; does your doctor address these issues when it comes to your medical condition? Can you get well without addressing these issues?

The studies that show the connection to good financial credit and better health have a solid basis in the internal focus. The same applies to studies showing that people with better relationships enjoy better health—again validating the internal focus.

COMPLETE BUSINESS PARADIGM

If we apply the same health paradigm and principles above to business or personal finances, we see that the business built to last has the common ground of the internal focus approach.

The disease-germ theory-healthcare model and principles, if applied to a business, sound outrageous. The news is filled with many stories of business being built on a house of cards and the resultant bankruptcy, failure, fraud, or deception.

When it comes to money or business, we must treat it in a similar way we treat our body: stewards or trustees respecting it for what it connects us with. Why do we need to take care of our body? Why do we need to take care of finances or the land? The Native Americans claim that no one owns the land and we are the caretakers.

We can have money and be poor or slave to it. We can have money attained through vice, and it will undoubtedly be fleeting. Hopefully, we can have money and be liberated.

I believe science can prove the connection between the attainment of money and keeping it versus the failure to manage money. The research must be based on the map outlined within, distinguishing between external and internal. If science uses the same premise of the medical germ theory, no light will be shed. Research has shown the connection between money and happiness, money and health, and money and relationships. My theory is that if you selected people in their 60's—who are in a satisfying marriage, are not in debt, and are not on any pharmaceutical medications—to pick stocks or make decisions for financial planning; you would see remarkable results.

The common sense approach to having money, attaining it or maintaining it would go like this: Your business is low on capital, or is struggling with sales; the CEO or owner blames the low capital or decrease in sales on the economy, bad luck, chance, untrustworthy dealings, etc.; the CEO looks for solutions that are external like borrowing money, cheating, fudging bank statements or suing someone. The above scenario leads to business failure. When a business faces pain (illness), how they respond is the predictor of success. The examples are many. The accountant fudges the books to prepare for the end of the quarter and if he doesn't make earning look higher than they are they lose investors or stock value. It is just a matter of time until the cards fall.

In the complete paradigm, the CEO internalizes the situation and looks for solutions that are internal. The CEO embraces the fact that other businesses face the same economic challenges in a down economy and it is up to them to respond by getting better or living up to the challenge. Ultimately the business has a purpose and vision of helping people and providing a win-win for their customers. If sales are low, instead of fudging the books for investors, it responds responsibly as a wakeup call to become leaner, more competitive, and more creative. In the short-term, it may be a setback or messy. In the long-term, the company stays whole.

The similarities between business and health, and relationships and health are remarkable. If you spend more than you make, chances are you will not embrace this paradigm. If you are in control and responsible for your finances, you most likely attribute the success to your intrinsic qualities and have a significantly better chance of embracing the same responsibility for your health. I have found clinically that my patients who are in control of their finances have greater success at healing than those who have money problems.

Drugs and treatments are so ingrained in our beliefs as acceptable and normal that people believe taking narcotics and masking the symptoms for their health problems is normal. In the healthy business arena CEOs do not take drug equivalents for their business pains. After reading and studying successful businesses, business leaders, and individuals that are financially solid, I found that they do not waiver nor opt for the shortcut or "drug" to mask symptoms or pain.

In the future, our society will look upon taking all drugs as being unacceptable, just as we are starting to do with cigarettes. At present some businesses reject the drugs (cheating and shortcuts) and take an internal framework instead.

The successful business model sees taking the shortcut/drug as painful. The CEO considers a temptation of temporary pain relief being outweighed by the pain of the cost of the shortcut. People who have money troubles take on the belief that money has to do with luck, chance or genetics. They believe that you have to be lucky, or born into money to have money. The opposite is true of people who have money—it has everything to do with being financially responsible.

My clinical experience is that people who are financially secure—not necessarily rich—are the people who are more open to heal and be healthy by looking inside. Clarifying your definition of wealthy versus rich is important. An interesting point is the proof that those with better credit scores have better health and higher life expectancy.

I enjoy working with financially secure people and especially enjoy working with financially successful people. They are more willing to not look for the shortcuts or to place blame on luck, chance or genetics. Their results with health are more consistent and quicker. Whenever the successful patient starts to give me a lot of 'yeah buts' we apply their resistance back to business and finances. In doing so, they quickly get back on track to using the solid foundation and principles. For someone who has not mastered self-control and responsibility with money, the challenge is more significant.

Some may think that those who spend the most on healthcare have the longest life expectancy. The same would apply to those who pay the most on pharmaceuticals. The reality is that the increased spending on healthcare and pharmaceuticals does not improve one's health or life expectancy. There is a much stronger correlation with those who have good to excellent credit reports having better health, along with those in healthy relationships.

COMPLETE RELATIONSHIP PARADIGM

The relationship is the single most crucial factor to our overall health and well-being. It is through the relationship that we become whole. It is through the relationship that we ultimately see ourselves change and heal. Like health and finances, relationships are governed by the same principles. Those in meaningful, purposeful, serving and loving relationships follow the internal/internal approach. The painful ones are equally important.

Financial health gives feedback that is more black and white. If your business fails you have no money; if you get fired from your job, you have no money. You can see from your monthly bank statements and credit cards if you are "off."*Blaming* forces people to choose between being right and being happy. Money is required for wants and needs. You may get your needs met by receiving welfare. For most people welfare is not acceptable and they respond with principle-centered action and figure out that blaming (externalizing) doesn't work. Our society is divided 80/20. We have people who have given up and live the external/external, while others have complete control of their finances, with solid work ethics and virtues, living internal/internal. We also have everything in between. Where are you on this continuum? Ask yourself why. The solution is found in your response.

When we see the cause and effect of our actions on health and relationships the timeline is significantly different. If you start to gain weight or increase your blood sugar levels, or your blood pressure is elevating... in the short term, so what! The only thing you may observe is that your energy is low. You react by drinking more coffee, or soda, and get clothes an extra size up. The problem is not pressing until you are obese, diabetic, or you have a heart attack. With relationships, the pain is also not immediate. We can blame, find fault, or be the victim or the jerk, and continue to function. We go from one unfulfilling relationship to the next. Many stay in dysfunctional "codependent" relationships because on the surface it is the path of least resistance.

In our relationships, emotions and feelings can get buried. By suppressing emotions, symptoms emerge and cause pain. I have found in my 20 plus years in practice that addictions and health problems are rooted in relationship conflict and suppressed emotions. There are several types of relationships: Your relationship with yourself (meaning you as a child, parent, worker, community member, team member, etc.); your relationship with your parents; your relationship with your spouse; your relationship with your children; your relationship with a close friend; your relationship with your community; your relationship with your health; your relationship with your money (meaning money you have, or don't have, overspending, savings, work and retirement).

Mastering your relationships requires virtues. To examine your relationship with your spouse, we see the same patterns. Here are three long-term predictors of divorce that the studies discovered: As you read through the following ask yourself if these patterns reflect an external/external approach or an internal/internal approach.

(The following is from a UCLA study) A lack of communication. Couples who divorced often used blame and invalidation when they communicated, while successful couples were more open and affirming. Even couples with drastically different opinions stayed together as long as they communicated well and supported each other.

The presence of discouraging and aggressive behavior. Couples that eventually divorced often discouraged their spouses from expressing their feelings or showed aggression during arguments early in their marriage.

Pessimism. Perhaps the most interesting, researchers found that pessimism can lead to bad marriages, and bad marriages can increase pessimism. Inappropriate pessimism was a predictor of divorce, both when it came to how a person felt about small arguments and how a person felt about their overall happiness in life.

Marriage expert John Gottman identified four relationship patterns that can doom a marriage: criticism, defensiveness, stonewalling, and contempt. When any of those patterns predominate during conflict resolution, the marriage is in trouble.

Criticism combined with pessimism is a road to marriage failure. Objective criticism aimed at resolving an issue is acceptable and encouraged in relationships.

Pessimism begets more pessimism until divorce seems inevitable. Can couples learn optimism? I believe they can shift from pessimistic to optimistic only by working on themselves and ultimately seeing their partner in a favorable light—because they stop projecting their problems upon their partner. Partners who have a knee-jerk pessimistic view of their partner's behaviors as an attack on themselves will have poor outcomes. The optimistic partner who sees their partner's negative actions in a different light will conversely have a different relationship outcome. For example, if your partner is late, the pessimist will see this as an attack and they will believe that the action was personal. This means they think that their partner intended to be late to hurt them, does not respect them, believes the behavior will continue forever and believes that this behavior shows that they can't trust their partner in other areas of their relationship. Conversely, the optimist doesn't feel hurt by their partner being late, gives them the benefit of the doubt and provides alternative reasons for them being late. It is about their partner's time management, or perhaps something outside their partner's control interfered, or maybe they stopped to help someone. They believe that it is an isolated episode; they believe that this does not interfere with their level of trust of their partner in other areas.

It comes down to seeing your partner in the best light. Research has shown that in cases where partners see their significant other with high regard, goodness, or they idealized the other the partner, they were happier in their relationship. It comes down to respect and more importantly self-respect.

It comes down to the projections we put forward. If we see good in our partner it is coming from our own goodness. If we see negative, the same applies. If you have trouble seeing the good and are pessimistic, you must address and heal your negative past experiences, feelings, and beliefs that create this reality.

In an interview with the L.A. Times, Lisa Neff, Director of The Austin Marriage Project at the University of Texas (Austin), she pointed out that while couples need a very realistic perspective in order to solve specific conflicts and support each other, they also benefit from "having a positive overall glow, that things will work out for the best and that my partner is really a good person." (Rebecca Hagelin)

Similarly, Gottman's research points out that, as important as good conflict resolution skills are, they are not the cure-all for a failing marriage. Why? Because 69 percent of conflict in a marriage is "perpetual," meaning that it's more a function of personality issues and competing needs than a specific problem. Couples need to negotiate those conflicts but, more importantly, they need to build friendship, foster intimacy, and discover shared meaning in their lives. In so doing, they can reignite their optimism about each other and their marriage.

While a pessimistic view of the other person and the marriage worsens the relationship, cultivating a positive mindset towards your spouse—focusing on their strengths and gifts—says Neff, "remind you of why you're in that relationship in the first place."

Values clarification and purpose are the foundation of change. In reality, health is secondary to relationships. The purpose of being healthy is to access your purpose and potential in your relationships.

If you are sick, tired, foggy, and drugged up, you can't access your true potential for love, or whatever else your purpose is. Life becomes a struggle. My personal health goal is not to live the longest; it is to live light, clear, relaxed, strong and full of energy. I want to access my meaningful relationships and experiences with no rock unturned. When I face death I want to face it gracefully and embrace it like birth.

In relationships, we often come across challenges. When we heal our relationships, we become whole. This happens when we change internally. (See The Course In Health Workbook)

A "cure" for relationship challenges may be infidelity to satisfy your loneliness or urges. The infidelity may satisfy your symptom but does nothing to make you whole. Our society is sadly starting to accept "cures" or "relief" in relationships. This type of cure is no different than a drug.

SECTION 3
EDUCATION AND VIRTUES - THE FOUNDATION

A college degree may add ten years to your lifespan according to a study published in *Health Affairs*. This research also showed that a lack of education—those not completing high school—had a life expectancy similar to those 60 years ago. This in contrast to the fact that many people, living a simple, virtuous life in perhaps the Mediterranean or Africa, add years to their lives with their non-indulgent, non-overstimulating life, with a diet, activity, and lifestyle exuding self-control with little to no education. Sometimes education and virtues are learned in culture and through the family and not necessarily in the school.

The base and footings of your healthcare are rooted in education and virtues (the rock). I think most people accept this, yet the significant obstacle is changing behaviors, habits, and beliefs. The Latin root of the word Doctor is Teacher. Doctors have historically failed at teaching their customers about health and illness. When doctors don't teach they prescribe and treat. The 'prescribing and treating' separate the doctor and customer. It is a perplexing situation that arises in distinguishing between the two forces of the treating doctor versus the teaching doctor.

The teaching doctors encourage the educated customer to ask the question *why*. With the treating doctor's focus being on external treatments and believing exclusively in luck, chance and genetics, they often do not even know of the factual connections to diet and exercise related to illness.

If I want to get better at golf or playing the piano, I may sometimes need the guidance of a teacher. If that teacher simply gave me a pill to learn to play better, I would be skeptical. In the real world, the teacher first explains some principles, then shows me, then encourages me to practice while giving me feedback.

If I want to get better at my health, I need to understand how I get sick or how I stay healthy. If your doctor is not educating you on health principles or giving you feedback he or she is not a teacher/doctor, just a physician.

When I learned how to play golf, I accessed some great coaches, and one thing that stood out is the equal playing field I was put on. I felt empowered and encouraged that I could master the sport. Within a year of playing, I got a hole in one. As I continued to play, I witnessed that my improvements in the game directly correlated with changing ineffective techniques with good ones. An interesting fact is that the majority of golfers do not improve after the first five years of playing. I believe this is mostly because they refuse to change bad habits.

When it comes to doctors as teachers, the customer/student is often made to feel like they are small, and that they could never understand the complexities of health. The separation tends to have the customer feel like he is at the doctor's mercy.

The irony is that in medieval Europe surgeons didn't have a university education and the physician at the time considered surgery to be below them. The red and white barber pole that still exists today signified the blood and bandage and the work performed. The point is that surgery is an art and should be left to those qualified and experienced, yet at the same time it is not a mystical gift imparted upon a select few of highly intelligent individuals. We look down upon the street drug dealers that prescribe the same pills the guys in white lab coats do.

The pharmaceutical industry is empowering customers with drug knowledge. Advertising protocols give customers the ability to self-diagnosis, learn side effects and do the work of the doctor. However, when doctors are asked "why do I need this drug?" the customer is not given an educated response. The educated response by the doctor would be "To cover up symptoms." The customer's response should be, "Isn't that bad?"

When doctors are asked why I got this condition, the typical response is we don't know why. That is just not true. The correct answer takes too long for the pressured physician. The factual connections to diet and lifestyle resulting in illness can't be ignored.

When the customer becomes educated and empowered they are faced with making changes in their approach to health.

What education does is build self-esteem and self-control. With these tools customers can make an intelligent decision—often staying away from hospitals and doctors. It is believed that virtues lead us to happiness and that the connection between virtues and health is undeniable. Virtues are gained through education, self-awareness, self-control, and purpose. They are then taught, learned, and evolved.

Education and virtues are not about knowing everything (or having a high IQ) and they are not about being perfect; they are about learning and living with a purpose. It is overcoming our worldly egos and choosing to be whole and healthy. The question, "How does a greedy person 'be' charitable?" is answered in the workbook.

Knowing that a good percentage of the time we will be off-course, we can acknowledge the offenses and redirect ourselves back on track.

We all have a purpose in life and values that surround that purpose. All purpose is rooted in the virtues.

Do not look negatively to the vice because in suffering the vice we reach virtues. A person who can walk through the vice feeling the pain can change their consciousness in the process.

According to Nietzsche, virtues suffer when there is no authority of values. That means that if you don't have a Grand Purpose we see self-indulgent, immediate gratification and the acceptance of subpar moral values as the norm. What is acceptable as moral today may have gotten you thrown in jail years ago. What is acceptable for diet today would have been admonished 40 years ago.

The pendulum shifting on values may serve to direct us not to focus on being good, right and perfect, rather be *non-judgmental* of our vices to allow ourselves to return to the virtues that lead to wholeness *gently*. (See The Course In Health Workbook Section 2)

Aristotle believed that if we regulate our desires either too much or too little, we create problems. Similar to exercise, if we don't move or exercise we develop problems as do those that exercise too much.

The individual character traits that make you unique are intertwined in your move to virtue. For example, if you are by nature a fearful person you set out to develop virtuous traits of courage. If you go too far with this, you may become harsh or rash by overcompensation, which in turn becomes a vice, while the surrendering or avoiding vice would be cowardice. It is often difficult to be able to rise above the fear instead of fighting it or running away or avoiding. Below is a chart of the balanced virtue weighed against the surrendering or deficient virtue compared to the overcompensating, extreme or excess. Both extremes are becoming a vice.

DEFICIENCY	VIRTUE/VALUE	EXCESS
FEAR/COWARD	COURAGE	HARSH/RASH
PROCRASTINATE/LAZY	AMBITIOUS	UNRELENTING
INCOMPETENT	COMPETENT	PERFECTION
DEPRIVATION	TEMPERANCE	GLUTTONY
SHAME	HUMILITY	PRIDE
SELF PITY	EQUAL	SUPERIORITY
VICTIM	PEACE	ABUSIVE/PERP
RESENTMENT/VICTIM	FORGIVING	PUNITIVENESS
INSINCERE/ DISGUST	HONESTY, PURITY	TEMPTATION
PASSIVE AGGRESSIVE	PATIENCE	VIOLENT WRATH
GUILT/ UNETHICAL	INTEGRITY/JUSTICE	CORRUPTION
DENIAL	HONEST	DISHONEST
SCARCITY	CHARITY	GREED
SELF SACRIFICE	FAIR	ENTITLEMENT
DEPENDENT	STRONG	CONTROLLING
DEFECTIVE	BALANCED	GRANDIOSE
SLOTH/LAZINESS	DILIGENCE	OBSESSIVE
LUST	UNWAVERING/FAITHFUL	CORRUPTION
ABANDONED/ALIENATE	CONNECTED	DEPENDENT
INDIFFERENCE	KINDNESS	JEALOUS
OVERLY HUMBLE	BALANCE- PRIDE	VAIN
FALSELY MODEST	TRUTHFUL	BOASTFUL
DISLOYAL	LOYALTY	UNTRUSTING
POVERTY	VALUE	COMPETITION
ADDICTION	LOVE	MATERIALISM

Take a step back and ask yourself if you worship any vice—directly or indirectly—by way of your actions (for example, the perfectionism, superiority, and grandiose of professional athletes). Professional athletes and especially the elite-of-the-elite have to, by definition, live the vice in order to move from competency to perfection and competitively be the best.

Furthermore, examine yourself regarding the grandiose, superiority, and perfection vices you may admire in the actors or actresses in Hollywood or Royalty. If you value the superiority of Royalty can you live the virtue of equality? By idealizing/idolizing royalty or famous people (superiority) you are possibly doing one of two things: 1) telling yourself that you are inferior (self-pity) or 2) telling yourself that you value superiority and inequality because you want to be superior. This is not to be confused with celebrating someone else's strengths or gifts while remaining neutral to them. If you worship famous people's perfection by their physical appearance, how does that affect the virtue of your confidence?

I have always been amazed how so many people yield and worship the vices or the uber-wealthy by celebrating their gluttony, superiority and/or greed. How people treat the wealthy like gods or as different from other people reveals that the vice is more important than the virtue.

If by your actions you celebrate and ironically "envy" the vice can you heal past that? The masses are brainwashing the masses that the vice is okay and celebrated, while at the same time telling us the virtue is important. You can't have both. The reason these dilemmas are addressed is that if you are living with such conflict and are unaware it doesn't matter how hard you try.

VICE TO VIRTUE

VIRTUES
INTERNAL
CONVERT
EXTERNAL

Many books, research, and studies show the connection between success, health, and virtues. Most people are aware of the virtues mentioned above, along with their vices. The challenge is first identifying and then questioning the many references that support the vice and substitute them with the virtue. Sounds easier said than done. The tools in the workbook lead us to the virtues of health and happiness.

Virtues evolve in us with self-awareness, self-control, our purpose and getting in touch with our feelings. Ultimately accessing self-awareness/control and purpose together lead us to the virtues that give us happiness. We are not born this way. What if your support system has not ripened or you have not learned to exercise virtues? The simple answer is to find virtuous people and references to create change. Like attracts like. It is a fact of nature. The common quote of 'opposites attracts' is not true. If you look at the physics—positive and negative poles line up and like attracts like. It is why relationships give the amazing potential for healing.

SECTION 4

CHANGE HAPPENS:
WHEN SELF-AWARENESS MEETS SELF-CONTROL WITH A FOCUS ON THE GRAND PURPOSE

Self-control is the secret of stress management. There are two components of stress management: 1) Mind/thought management and 2) Body/physical management. The mind and body are inseparable but for ease of explanation, we will dissect them.

The body part of stress management is our physical well-being. Our ability to effectively handle stress is determined by our physical state. Our physical state is comprised of body chemistry which is caused by diet. Diet consists of air, water, food, or anything consumed. When these areas are balanced we are able to handle situations more effectively. To illustrate this let us take two different scenarios. Situation #1. Last night you got drunk, then woke up late for work and were rushed to eat breakfast. You had to race to work or face being late... again. Someone carelessly cut you off on the road. Chances are good you would respond with anger or fear—magnified. Situation #2. Last night you went to bed early. You got up in time to do exercise, stretching, prayer or meditation. You ate a balanced breakfast and then left for work early. Someone carelessly cut you off on the road. This time you barely glanced his way and continued on.

Mind/thought management has to do with how we interpret situations. When it comes down to it, it is not the stress but how we *react* to it that makes all the difference. Two people can be in identical situations and respond in totally different styles. Our personal interpretation of the situation makes a big difference. When we ask a different question of ourselves, we get a different answer. Our physical state combined with our mental state determines how we respond.

I would like to share a dialogue I had with a patient. He had come in for some neck problems. He related to me that his former physician (chiropractor) had not satisfied him. He understood the triad of health, or thought he did (physical, structural and emotional) and that was why he came to me. I explained how the foods we eat play a profound effect on muscles, along with breathing and water consumption. During his second visit for an adjustment, he asked me "What causes this neck pain? My last chiropractor said the vertebra was out and it is interfering with the nerve." So I explained to him that muscles move bones. In other words, muscle tension may cause the bone to go out of place. He replied, "So the real cause of my neck pain is muscle tension?" I then asked him what causes the muscle tension. He replied, "I get it. It's stress that causes the muscle tension, that causes the bone to go out of place, that irritates the nerve, that causes the pain." He almost had it. I asked him what is the difference between two people reacting completely differently in a similar situation. I.e. the reason your neck muscles are stiff is that your boss yelled at you. How can it be then that your co-workers received the same tongue-lashing and shrugged it off with no resulting muscle tension?

Neck pain results from any stressful situation put upon the structures affecting the neck, and include nutrition, toxins, muscle tension, stress, trauma, etc. This client ultimately did reach the answer he was seeking by merely changing the question he was asking.

There is no doubt that self-control is a large part of the foundation of our health. Be it relationship health, physical health or financial health. This 'self-control' with a clear purpose in life determines if we exercise, overeat, spend too much, save too little, commit to relationships, etc. We would all love to enjoy the self-control that leads us to regular exercise and optimal foods, along with positive choices in all areas of our life.

The double-edged sword: Any stress that we are exposed to will decrease our self-control. This happens because stress will temporarily reduce the blood glucose in your brain. People crave sugars or carbohydrates when they are stressed because they have low blood glucose in their brain. Sugars include bread, soda, alcohol, grain, etc.

Some drink excess alcohol when they are stressed. When you are intoxicated with alcohol the blood glucose in your brain is minimal, and people lack self-control.

The alcohol, which is a temporary stress reliever because it is a depressant, becomes a double-edged sword. It will do the job of temporary stress relief, however, the cost to this temporary stress relief in the form of physical body harm and a lack of self-control will put most in a negative balance.

Low blood glucose = low self-control
Increased stress = low blood sugar
Stress is unavoidable. Excess stress is mostly avoidable.

When we are stressed virtues are potentially compromised. Stress can be sleep deprivation, poor diet, over-stimulating foods or drugs, depleting foods or drugs, lack of exercise, electromagnetic stress, along with mental-emotional stress.

You need glucose in your blood to feed your brain to be able to exert self-control, and when you do exercise self-control, you burn glucose, which in turn makes it harder to exert self-control in the future. Amazing when physiology is applied to the real world.

SELF-ESTEEM AND SELF-WORTH

People with positive self-esteem/worth are more apt to exercise, succeed academically, question authority, make changes, and have healthy boundaries in relationships. Simply because they love and accept themselves they have an internal focus versus an external focus.

Low self-esteem has been shown to contribute to many health problems including depression, obesity, anorexia nervosa, bulimia, higher risk of suicide, and addictive behaviors.

Self-esteem must be balanced with a neutral optimistic and pessimistic point of view. It can become dangerous and misguided to build someone's self-esteem on areas that are not warranted.

By taking the virtues mentioned above and applying self-esteem or autonomyalong with a balanced approach to interpreting any event, situation, goal, or relationship, we can heal. We are not going to be able to experience all the virtues all the time. We are not going to fake it or pretend.

In the workbook, we take the virtues, self-control, self-esteem, combined with different beliefs and feelings, and incorporate them into a realistic, optimistic or pessimistic assessment of the event or condition. Sounds complicated but the exercise is simple.

"The man who does not value himself, cannot value anything or anyone."
—Ayn Rand, The Virtue of Selfishness

"Nothing builds self-esteem and self-confidence like accomplishment."
—Thomas Carlyle

"The experience of being competent to cope with the basic challenges of life and being worthy of happiness." —Nathaniel Branden

BALANCE - NOT MODERATION

To understand a balanced approach to healthcare we need to step back and appreciate the dualist approach to life which is the explanation of two opposing and complementary forces coming together as ONE. From a philosophical sense it may identify material matter versus the mental, while from the biblical viewpoint, it may look at the body versus the soul.

Never explain dualism as good and evil. Instead, it is about opposing and connecting/complementary forces. Day and night, east and west, in and out, heaven and earth. (Complete list below) There is no finite day or night; instead each flow into each other, just as east and west do. Our beings (body and soul) consist of the same flow between spiritual and earthly. The spiritual part is about our purpose and connection with a higher power. Our earthliness is our body, our environment and how we interact with it. The huge leap is how they connect. Day turns into night at dusk; then night turns into the day at dawn. We can see that no finite line separates day and night. In the west coast there is an east side of the beach and west side, and again on the west side of the beach, there is an east side and a west side, making the whole connected.

The one thing that has intrigued me since I was a teenage boy watching the stars is the concept of infinity. I don't claim to have a grasp of the full concept—yet I will continue to ask the questions. I believe the concept of infinity has led me to my questions and my receiving some answers to health. I think that infinity and connection to our universe and the concept of a dualistic approach will shift one's thinking and lead to healing. Getting in touch with our masculine and feminine dualism—right and left brain— and physical body and soul (or spirit) is where I believe healing begins.

The problem is that we have made medicine "masculine," and it is not working. Let's look at other professions and agree that they are either mostly masculine or feminine, while only some are balanced. Feminine means they are more about timelessness, connection, nurture, feelings, etc. versus masculine meaning mathematical, logical, timely, etc. The first profession that comes to mind is accounting. It is mostly black and white and mathematical—making it a masculine profession. We can all agree that when masculine qualities prevail we succeed in this profession—our taxes are done correctly and on time. Not much room for feelings and nurture needed in accounting firms. At the same time, abstract thinking and the feminine side help on the creative side of accounting. Great accountants respect the masculine qualities and also embrace that one plus one can equal any number with creativity. Let's agree that accounting exudes 80 percent masculine and 20 percent feminine.

The daycare business: The daycare business is about nurturing and providing a healthy environment for children. The successful daycare will embrace mostly feminine qualities including warmth, creativity, nurture, yet still needs the masculine attributes of time for pick up/drop off feeding schedules, etc.

We can analyze each profession and see that all professions must have both masculine and feminine qualities. Relationships are the same way. Strong masculine men attract strong feminine women. It is a balancing act. More feminine men attract more masculine women.

Our medical system is 98-100 percent masculine with less than two percent feminine coming from nurses and chaplains. The data and research clearly show that medicine only helps eight to 20 percent of conditions, yet continues to use the masculine approach for the 80 percent plus of conditions it cannot help.

Please don't confuse doctors trying desperately to connect more and show more compassion by spending more time with patients, or trying to be "spiritual" then going right back to the disconnect of external cause/external cure. They are in the business of selling drugs and treatments, not being spiritual or feminine. The same wolf in sheep's clothing exists in natural medicine, posing as spiritual then separating you by giving you pills, treatments and making the "healer" or doctor be an "all-knowing guru." Beware of any person who calls themselves a healer. Physician... heal thyself.

Masculine Professions: Tech, accounting, law, law enforcement, fireman, sports media, math, physics, politics, construction. Why is it that over 98 percent of all roofers, mechanics, concrete workers, and loggers are men? Why are over 92 percent of all childcare workers, receptionists, secretaries, assistants, dental hygienists, dental assistants, and speech pathologists women?

I am not in any way questioning or suggesting that the predominant professions of women change gender roles by saying we need more men in daycare or more women roofers or diesel mechanics. I believe it would be a mistake.

I do believe that if we changed the focus/map from masculine dominance to feminine dominance in healthcare we would actually start to see healing as the norm. The areas where females would excel are politics, law, and medicine. I am not suggesting that we need more women in politics, law, and medicine acting like men. This would be a disaster. I am suggesting we allow women to bring their strengths to these professions and watch how things change for the better. I am also suggesting that until we realize that these systems are built on sand, we will continue to spin our wheels.

Many of the problems or challenges faced by politicians, judges, lawyers, and doctors require both right and left brain thinking. If you don't think that politics and law are a spiritual process, ask yourself if you believe that judges, lawyers, and politicians are helping world peace or creating war? If the judge (woman or man) is driven by power and masculine forces it leads to the corruption we see in our legal system. Payoffs and bribes are the norms with masculine form.

The problem is that these professions that have been set up and ruled by men, have not been challenged from their inception. The fix is not just pushing women into the model without fixing the map. These professions started at the same time that the same men believed the world was flat. We changed the map and rules regarding the world being flat—we can now sail around the world— so the world is now connected as a result. We have not addressed the elephant in the room: the old masculine thinking that governs politics, law, and medicine. This is not about separation of church and state. It is re-establishing our map on these failed systems.

Much of the information provided in this book is about shifting to the feminine side for balance. There is no question that our medical system is a strongly masculine-directed force. Like accounting and law professions they are black and white professions. Accounting, medicine, and law have historically been male professions. Historically women have not been attracted to the masculine type of profession that requires mathematics and science. There is no need for debate that women are equally capable in any profession.

Healthcare is not black and white. If your doctor does not understand the dualist approach to health, the chances are good he or she is giving you bad advice. The lopsided fact is that our medical system is all about the so-called new and improved treatment of the pill approach, giving all credit to the procedure.

Typically women are wired to be nurturing while men usually are wired to be the breadwinners. Many women and men excel in either area. The balance of masculine and feminine attributes and qualities is necessary. It doesn't mean that the woman who has the strong desire to stay home needs to prove herself by excelling in the workforce. If there are imbalances in masculine and feminine energies, they must be addressed.

The paradigm and information provided here is geared towards rebalancing the medical system. There are strengths and positives to the masculine side of our medical system. These are the areas where medicine works and requires respect. Emergency medicine and the 20 percent of treatments and prescriptions that are used to buy time or offer a cure need to be respected. As a doctor who sees a wide array of conditions and teaches many effective ways to treat conditions I can say that the same percentages for effective treatment in acupuncture, chiropractic, and supplementation are effective and many conditions will resolve and heal with time, stress management and internal means. I believe 80 percent of what is presented in a doctor's office would resolve with a feminine medical model. A chiropractor adjusting a patient who has suffered from headaches for years is similar to the MD setting a bone to allow for healing to take place.

The balance between masculine and feminine—or yin and yang—can be thought of as complementary and not opposing forces. Everything has both masculine and feminine qualities. One of the most critical aspects of this balance is that masculine and feminine both require the other for their existence.

In eastern medicine the qualities of masculine and feminine are explained as yin and yang.

Yin	**Yang**
Female	Male
Night	Day
Moon	Sun
Low	High
Heavy	Light
Falling	Rising
Inward	Outward
Interior	Exterior
Front	Back
Left Side	Right Side
Acid	Alkaline
Right Brain	Left Brain
Timelessness	History
Non-logical	Logical
Tonal	Mathematical
Non-Sensible Abstract	Rational
Unpredictable	Reasonable
Parasympathetic	Sympathetic
Slow	Fast

Soft	Hard
Wet	Dry
Cold	Hot
Passive	Aggressive
Soul	Body

Notice that cure and healing, and good or bad, are not a part of this! We are often mistaken by the concept of yin and yang, somehow attributing them as opposites and somehow incorporating good and evil in the same sentence. They are opposing yet connecting qualities. The concept of "opposite" is in essence of "similarity" in which these factors are always bound together, intertwined as a whole, where one can't exist without the other. For example, we can't have the day without night; we can't have a palm of a hand without having the back of the hand. The same can be said of Love and Hate. Nor could we have men without women. The cycle of life is found within this concept.

The five elements of LIFE are Wood, Fire, Earth, Metal, and Water. There is a constructive cycle: Wood feeds Fire - Fire creates Earth (ash) - Earth creates Metal - Metal enriches Water - Water feeds Wood.

There is a destructive cycle: Wood can break the ground (Earth) - Earth can soak up or block Water - Water puts out Fire - Fire can melt Metal - Metal cuts Wood.

The breathing exercises in the workbook are intimately connected to the "Balance." The breathing exercises are an essential exercise with access to both Masculine and Feminine.

We can see an orderly, purposeful cycle of constructive and destructive cycles reflective in nature and our lives. A study of the excess or deficiency in these elements leads back to creating balance. This is no different from the lifecycles of animals in the wild: Birds, fish, deer, and wolves all need each other. When one is taken out, an imbalance occurs. The reintroduction of wolves into Yellowstone showed how the wolves being repopulated helped the rivers, bison, and birds.

Too much focus on one aspect of your life, (for example work, money or partying) will probably lead to illness in another area. The cycle and corrections help restore the balance.

Not respecting this balance will always lead to illness. I have clinically seen these correlations with patients over the last 20 years. Often I see the feminine quality of the yin with patients being carefree with time and appointments. These people are usually late. Some may see this as a strong positive yin quality that allows for patience and relaxation. The flip side is that this beautiful feminine quality may cause problems in their life. The opposite would hold true of the masculine quality of mathematical, logical, and time where the person is always on time, has a balanced checking account, and obsesses over lists. This may cause rigidity and cause more stress than benefit. If any of these energies are off, they cause problems. If the problems (imbalance) cause illness, understanding the connection is the foundation of change.

The cycles of up and down and life and death happen continuously. Our whole existence can be compared to waves in the ocean.

One way to address this is to look at life as an expression of happiness and death as an expression of sadness. To take a step back and realize that death creates life and in life, death ensues.

Success and failure are normal; it is a fantasy to expect only success. We are taught that we should only expect pleasure without pain. This creates a significant confusion surrounding health AND PAIN.

If we can't embrace the feminine side or masculine side, we then can't embrace pleasure because of the avoidance of pain. Sounds deep but it isn't. Simply put, if you are unable to embrace your dark side, physical pain, or your painful emotional past, it is not possible to create the balance of your "light."

Let me clarify the embracing of the feminine side. Some people do not tolerate abstract thinking, timelessness, or the artistic side which partly describes the attributes of feminine energy. Some people do not tolerate masculine energy. It has been said that healing takes place when the right brain connects with the left brain.

Imbalanced right brain dominance is said to lead to religious fanaticism; they may have victim-mentality and generally believe that they need to rely on a "god" or authority (doctor) to heal them.

Imbalanced or dominant left brain dominance is said to lead to too much logic and science, often leading to black and white thinking lacking creativity, natural understanding, spiritual awareness and intuitive skills. We need the balance of the right brain. "Science without religion is lame, religion without science is blind." —Albert Einstein.

The desire of all optimism and no pessimism, or no pain and all pleasure, leads to this disconnect from left and right brain. This is what our medical system is doing with pain. It's obsessed with avoiding pain. Embracing pain with feminine qualities allows for healing—it's not being a martyr. If you think so ask yourself if your child should experience the "pain" of delayed gratification or if there is a virtue in "painful" waiting. In the workbook, we address these imbalances. Receiving and giving bring about wholeness, while imbalances create illness.

So what does the feminine/masculine balanced medical system look like? First, we must embrace that healing is an internal process, and without respecting this feminine side, healing eludes us. Second is the aspect of our health that is external and relies on earthly things like diet or exercise and sometimes external medical or natural treatments. The imbalance is the focus on the external.

We need to accept that illness and pain are goal-oriented and purposeful. When our child falls to his knees and comes crying in pain, most often he needs to be held and loved. He doesn't need aspirin, ibuprofen or arnica. In talking with ER nurses, oncology nurses and doctors, and everyone in between, the feminine observation and opinion are that these visits are just about people needing love and reassurance. The only thing that our medical system offers is a lot of compassion with very little empowerment. We come to the clinic or hospital to be touched, heard and loved and then we are given pills to cover the pain.

When you bring your car in for a brake job, all you want is a precise masculine form of service. When you bring your kids to daycare, you don't want them treated like a car. You want nurturing, listening, patience, etc. When we go to doctors and clinics, we are often treated like a car. So what is the solution? Stop trying to put the square peg into the round hole. Stop trying to heal by going to doctors. You go to a surgeon, and your problem is you need surgery. You go to a psychiatrist, and your problem is you are in need of prescription medication. You go to an acupuncturist and you need needles put in specific locations.

I don't want the message I deliver to be that these professions are bad—I am not saying that. If you go for the masculine treatment, you get masculine treatment. You can't complain about the chemotherapy or prescription causing problems when you asked for that treatment. It goes back to blaming the McDonald's for making you fat and tired when the deeper reality is that McDonald's did exactly what it was set out to do: make the shareholder's money, not produce health. The meds and treatments have a specific goal: to separate you from pain.

Hopefully, this section is not confusing but thought-provoking. I am saying that our medical system needs to change and at the same time saying we have allowed and created this system. There are many aspects of our medical system that are off, and at the same time, medical doctors seldom talk about healing and almost always discuss their approach as a cure. It is honest. We the consumer do not discern the difference. Can you explain the difference between healing and a cure? Do you want the symptoms to go away? Or do you want to heal? Huge difference!

The same applies to the side effects of drugs and surgery. For the most part, the nasty, harmful side effects are given to the consumer—listen to the TV commercials or read the magazine advertisements. They are honest.

If the earth was the center of the universe 300 years ago, we don't need to blame the people who made the claim or the people who believed it. We just need to move forward and stop the insanity of believing something that is not true. The same applies to our medical beliefs. They are not correct. We continue to believe them when the proof is that the earth is not the center. The leap is looking *inside* for healing and seeing the results.

Roger Bannister led the way to break barriers and limiting beliefs with running. I want to help in breaking the barriers to health and healing. The complexities I put forward are a balanced approach to healthcare. Looking at religions like the Christian Scientists that don't allow for any medical procedures is a drastic approach to incorporating the feminine side of health. I respect and honor many of the beliefs by their approach yet question the lack of accepting the masculine side of the medical system in the small percentage of cases. Again we can't treat our bodies like cars and at the same time, we can't go off the deep-end and not respect the mechanical and physical side of our bodies.

Ask questions about the circle of life and death, and you will then start seeking something beyond it. Through birth and death, we can learn so much about the life in-between.

THE DUALIST APPROACH TO INTERNAL VS. EXTERNAL

"There seems to be no plan because it's all a plan. There seems to be no center because it's all center." —C.S. Lewis

Why do we exercise? Some may exercise to help a medical condition or reduce weight. This is an external focus in exercise. Why others exercise is because they love the process of the activity; it gives them joy or they feel peace while engaging in the activity or they connect with friends in the activity or with nature while hiking, etc. These are focused on an internal drive.

Exercise with an external focus is detrimental because of the emotions that focus on fear, shame, disease, etc. This has an adverse effect on your physiology. Why do you think that some people doing exercise get benefits and others do not? People get positive side effects from exercise when their focus is internal. You *can* still get results with an external focus like in bodybuilding or the runner wanting to lose weight. The challenge is whether it's lasting or causes injury or another side effect to your psyche. This can be confusing because we can also look at two people running a marathon. During a marathon you will burn about 3000 calories – doesn't matter if your focus was internal or external. The dualist understanding of internal versus external can be explained. Smoking cigarettes kills the squamous cells in your respiratory system but how can some smoke for 50 years and not develop cancer? The answer is in the dualist understanding. For the runner completing the marathon for internal reasons they will more likely not get injured, and they will have an internal sense of well-being versus the tension or muscle stress associated with doing the marathon for external reasons like weight loss or approval seeking. To explain: If your focus is external while running you most likely will have high cortisol levels associated with your subconscious thoughts (high cortisol is a stress hormone causing breakdown). If the focus is internal while running (i.e., a happy Forest Gump runner) you will have high growth hormone levels (high growth hormone is the anti-aging hormone). The difference in physiological outcomes is measurable.

Consider food. Why do we see so many vegans and vegetarians who are sickly? Why do we see drastic changes in people's medical issues when they change their diet from pesticide to organic or processed to natural? The dualist approach applies. Wholefood diets are proven to produce better health; so why does changing one's diet to a healthy one not provide the healing we desire all the time? The simple answer is if the food is focused on the external it will not do what it is intended to do. If the focus of the diet is to reduce blood pressure, kill cancer cells or reduce weight, the external focus will not allow for the healing. Put another way: One cannot simultaneously prepare for war and peace at the same time. The focus is the outcome. If the focus is cancer (Kill/War) the outcome is cancer. If the focus is changing to your Grand Purpose (a higher power/unity) then the foods will do what they are intended to do.

Therapeutic fasting is a remarkable medical tool. The result from fasting for so many medical conditions is indisputable and amazing. I call it the fastest way to healing. One of the most obvious benefits is for blood pressure. All cases of hypertension end after an extensive fast. The majority of cases, when hypertension returns, are the result of old patterns. The doctors facilitating the fast will blame the return of high blood pressure on food (external). The fact is that it is and it isn't. For the answer, we can jump to the people healing from cancer with or without drastic dietary changes or fasting. If it was the diet how do we explain the person in remission that made no dietary changes? I propose that again the common denominator is on the focus and change that occurred in the remission: a focus on internal versus external. Does it mean food doesn't matter? NOT what I am saying. We cannot ignore the old belief in the germ theory and how the internal environment is critical in understanding.

I am saying that you don't need to exercise and still be healthy; I am saying that you don't need to eat organic and still be healthy; I am saying that you don't need to eat whole foods and still be healthy, etc. At the same time, the positive associations of these behaviors undoubtedly enhance your health. Furthermore, virtues lead you to a balanced diet and exercise. It's not hypocritical even though at the same time I'm making the claim that organic, wholefoods aid in health and healing. The differentiation is to not make food your religion.

I am saying that if exercise is external it will interfere with true healing and will not give sustaining results. I am saying that if food is external it will interfere with true healing. You will do the diet and maybe get results but the results are not sustaining.

Common sense dictates: do the things that are proven effective to improve your well-being. The catch is ONLY doing them with an internal focus. The next leap is how to make the focus internal; the simple answer is to have a purpose of belief in a higher power (see workbook).

If you exercise, diet, fast, and/or give up an addiction, the only way to achieve lasting results and whole health or healing is to do it out of love or pleasure or The Grand Purpose. When we do it to avoid pain, pain becomes the focus, and that's what we get.

The next leap is your willingness to change. This may mean addressing your addiction and vice. With changing, you may need to—or better yet be compelled to—start being more physically active or changing your diet.

One of the most significant external focuses in many people's lives is the attainment of medical services for healing. The belief and focus that the doctor, god, guru or a pill "fixed you" is fundamentally flawed. One of the major objectives of this book is to address this madness. I believe external-based medicine (natural and mainstream) is one of the single most significant impediments to healing. One of the most substantial challenges we face today is the pervasive (widespread) belief of external focus on medicine. Our medical system strives to be gods that separate you from healing. The goal of healthcare follows the same principles of internal versus external.

If we believe in the internal focus principle for relationships, wealth, and exercise, how can we exempt food and medicine from the same principle? I don't believe we can.

I propose that illness is a subconscious manifestation of our separation with our whole self. When the subconscious believes in the external we create illness to direct us back to unity.

External forces have hijacked our subconscious. These include the television shows we watch, from the actual show to the commercials, which create separation with our subconscious. The many other examples of our subconscious being hijacked are overwhelming. Our medical system has hijacked the subconscious equal to or more than TV, Hollywood, advertising, media, etc.

The process of the well-intentioned doctor directing people to health with an external treatment really makes healing difficult. This can be compared to me telling a patient that magnesium chelate is helpful for migraines, ovarian cysts, or menstrual cramping, etc. (As well as the adjustment for a headache, the acupuncture for the carpal tunnel syndrome and the medical antibiotic treatment for sepsis). Because the focus was on taking this for that, the subconscious is pushed to separation. There needs to be a shift in the delivery of the message from the doctors explaining the difference between curing and healing.

So when the patient gets lasting results—or healing—is it the result of the treatment or in spite of it? If you can't possibly prepare for war and peace at the same time, how can you possibly fight illness and create peace? If the focus of attaining health is through peace does this ONE THING bring about lasting healing? I believe so. This explains how some can heal cancer without changing diet or exercise, or how some can smoke cigarettes their entire life and not develop illness. At the same time when your focus changes to an internal one the probability of wanting to smoke or eat poorly diminishes. You subconsciously eat and exercise not because you want to rid a condition, rather because you love yourself. The war on "disease" or "addiction" cannot lead to healing. This might produce relief or cure—not healing.

Please be aware of your level of resistance with the preceding. It's big. All natural and mainstream medical focuses on avoiding pain. In this focus the failure is pervasive. The hypocrisy is that both medicines require fear and separation to gain control of the customer. It will drive you away from healing.

In spite of the fact that most natural and allopathic medicine sabotages healing and focuses on the magic of temporary cures, we can only step back and ask: is the medicine (natural and allopathic) as crazy a belief as the earth being the center of the universe? In fact, it is! If medicine were valid and scientific, it would work. Why we accept procedures, surgeries, drugs, pills, and acupuncture that mostly do not work or cause significant side effects is because it allows us to live in an illusion of separation or it gives temporary relief. Why would anyone choose separation over unity? This has been the biblical and philosophical question of man forever. I think Marianne Williamson says it best: "It's our light, not our darkness that we are most afraid of." In our journey of growth and change, we can use illness to unite or to link our purpose to our virtues.

If you still believe in the natural and medical model do you consider loan sharking or payday loans, or increasing credit card limits to be the answer to your money problems? They are short-term cures to money problems. They make the symptoms go away, yet be sure... they will return.

OPTIMISTIC VS. PESSIMISTIC VS. REALIST

"If you can own your hero and your villain, your saint and
your sinner, your two sides equally, you don't need nature to
have to get you back into balance. Those who can't govern
themselves attract events to govern them." —Nietzsche

Our internal filters of events determine how we respond to situations or events. For simplicity, we can say that events are positive, negative or neutral or better yet purposeful. The goal is to achieve autonomy, self-control and healthy self-esteem in events that come into our lives. The following is a cognitive basis for understanding how we interpret events in our lives and how to change. The serenity quote best applies: "God grant me the serenity to accept the things I cannot change, the courage to change the things I can, and the wisdom to know the difference." (Reinhold Niebuhr)

What this means for the following work is that certain beliefs, thoughts, and feelings are making us sick. We are asking for the courage to change these limiting beliefs, thoughts, experiences and use empowering words to make a change.

When a positive event happens in your life you can respond as if the event was attributed to you and your positive qualities, or impersonal—not having to do with you but instead more about other factors. You also consciously or subconsciously see the event as permanent or temporary. Lastly, we see the event as pervasive or specific. When a negative situation occurs we address the event with the same filters. Filters of events determine how we respond to situations or events.

Pervasive means spreading through every part of the issue. Typically an optimist will perceive—through thought, words, feelings, and beliefs—that a positive event is permanent and pervasive. The optimist will also perceive negative events as temporary and specific. The opposite holds true for the pessimist.

Many sick states are a result of inaccurate assessments of events of our life. The pattern continues until the pain becomes loud enough for us to change.

All addiction is the byproduct of our unfulfilled highest values. Addiction is looking for immediate gratification when we are not feeling fulfilled in our life; the compensation makes us feel more volatile. It makes us sick.

If you have the power from inside, you don't need external power. That is why much of the political system is off. If the people in power come from a place of internal power they have little or no need for external power and control. If the power comes from external then politicians can be bought for a price.

In the workbook, the imbalance of pessimistic and optimistic is addressed. One challenge is the forced optimistic thoughts that are overshadowed by pessimistic words and beliefs. Trying to be optimistic while you are ill is very problematic; it causes more illness. The challenging (radical) exercises allow us to demonstrate and change.

SECTION 5
IT'S NOT MAGIC. WHAT'S IN THE PILL?

Often I will ask my customers how the medication or pill works that they are putting in their body. I don't believe that I have ever been provided a good answer. Usually I get "Don't have a clue" or "I have never asked" responses. The simple answer I am looking for is: This drug is doing what my body is not doing at this time. Our body can produce analgesics (pain meds) better than any drug. If your body can't, there is a reason—a reason that is mostly or wholly ignored.

I explain that it is not necessary to understand the physiology and biochemistry in the pharmaceutical—it is, however, necessary to ask if the pill is magic or just chemicals made in a lab that mimic your own body's neurotransmitters, hormones, etc. This will set the stage for more questions on cause and effect.

The pill is given externally to provide your body with something that it's not able to produce or manufacture internally at that time.

WHAT IS HEALTH?

The World Health Organization (WHO) defines health as "a state of complete physical, mental, and social well-being and not merely the absence of disease or infirmity."

What is literacy? For most people, they simply define it as the ability to comprehend written and verbal language. However, many urged that the definition of literacy be expanded to include the ability to comprehend computer symbols, along with written music with the scope of this definition. Bottom line: One word can mean something different depending on one's personal or cultural standards.

When it comes to your health, consider raising your bar and expanding your definition of health to include your relationships, your finances, and your physical health, along with defining cure, relief, and healing.

For me, to be healthy is to experience all of the following:

To have superb energy levels throughout the day, allowing for the body's normal rhythm of activity and rest. To have peace, balance, and harmony in all areas of your life—spiritual health, financial health, social, career, contribution, and mental-emotional health. To enjoy deep and restful sleep at night. To have flexibility and strength. To be in the process of supreme health is to have no need to criticize others or to feel hurt yourself. It is to realize that our behavior stems either out of love or out of a need for love. To realize that every human being was once a beautiful, innocent, loving baby who may or may not have experienced abundant love and support while growing.

To be healthy is to understand that the gifts of life are for service, not for self-indulgence. It is to understand that the surest way to be happy is to make others happy. It is to realize that our needs are always met. Our unlimited potential to contribute flourishes when we rise above the survival mode and begin expressing our gratitude through our attitude. To be healthy is to wake up each morning with a sense of joy and gratitude. To make the most of each interaction in our relationships, and to live in each moment. The physical things described above are a natural consequence of the mind and body being at peace.

WHAT IS DISEASE? IS IT ILLNESS?

An illness is an abnormal condition that affects the mind or body of an organism. In humans, "Disease" is often used more broadly to refer to any condition that causes pain, dysfunction, distress, social problems, or death to the person.

WHAT IS FAILURE? WHAT IS SUCCESS?

Failure is the state or condition of not meeting a desirable or intended objective, and may be viewed as the opposite of success.

"I've failed over and over and over again in my life and that is why I succeed." —Michael Jordan

"Failure is success if we learn from it." —Malcolm S. Forbes

We take the two above quotes and substitute failure and success with illness and healing:
"I've gotten sick over and over and over again in my life and that is why I've healed."
"Illness is healing if we learn from it."

If Success comes from Good judgment...
If Good judgment comes from Experience...
If Experience comes from Poor judgment...

We must take our "poor judgment" and be gentle and optimistic to turn it into an experience that leads us to success. Poor judgment can lead to illness or failure when we are hard on ourselves or react in negative ways as to not gain "experience" from the poor judgment.

Being overweight, having high blood pressure, having high blood sugar, cancer or a cold is just the reality of our poor judgment or a call to heal. They purposefully help to guide us back to health. We ultimately thank and embrace the poor judgment gently. We then heal.

IS ILLNESS A MISTAKE OF NATURE?

Making mistakes gives us constant feedback, and when this feedback is taken with healthy beliefs, we take mistakes or failures and create success. Many people's lives are full of references or examples of succeeding through failure. When it comes to school, sports, work, and finances most of us get it. We learn how to swing a golf club or baseball bat largely by the "mistakes" that give the feedback to learn to become successful. In business, we do the same. However, there is a disconnect with our health. Most people do not see illness as a goal-oriented failure. Most people see and have been taught that illness is a mistake that we are victim to.

Is illness a mistake of nature? A careful study of the illness process reveals the incredible wisdom of the body, and it's never ending instinct to be well. We must remind ourselves that sniffles, aches, pains, and discomfort are important messages that we can choose to listen to. Consider what you do when the fire alarm goes off at work. Do you rip the alarm off of the wall, or stuff cotton balls in your ears? My guess is that you do neither. You look for the fire, put it out, and work on ways to prevent future fires. All signs and symptoms are messages from your body in the hopes that you will listen and make the changes that are necessary to reveal your health.

Have you ever had diarrhea? A runny nose? Hives? Cough? These are your body's first attempts to keep your body clear of toxins. Do you know anyone with heartburn? An ulcer? Skin rash? Chronic ear infection? Painful urination/bladder infection? These are some of the conditions that represent the body's next line of defense, using "inflammation" as a focused attempt to eliminate toxins and restore health. How about someone with cysts? Polyps? Red, hot, swollen areas? This person is losing a great deal of energy as she deals with the continuing build-up of toxins and is slowly becoming weaker on all fronts. High blood pressure, adult-onset diabetes, thyroid disease, kidney disease, heart disease and ultimately cancer are all states of breakdown, brought about by extreme toxic burden and weakened defenses.

What about insufficiency and deficiency conditions? For example, vitamin A, B or C deficiencies. A recent study showed that over 80 percent of North Americans were low in the RDA levels of at least one nutrient. This is attributed to a complex combination of circumstances. Many of the foods Americans eat are nutrient depleted and are full of empty calories. Another factor that contributes to deficiencies is overindulgence and stimulants. Overindulgence can be eating too much of one food, eating foods that are too rich, or eating certain foods in the wrong combination. Any of the above scenarios can cause your reserve of digestive enzymes to be depleted. Enzymes are crucial for every single function of the body, from seeing, to thinking, to moving, immune function, hormone production, etc.

Stimulants also leach out nutrients. The four stimulants I will discuss are virtually identical in their destructive aspect to the body. They are coke, tobacco, coffee, and cocaine. These stimulants require vitamins, minerals and other nutrients for the body to process and excrete them. When they are taken into your system, your body will subsequently release chemicals (catecholamines, for instance). This is the chemical explanation for the sense of well-being that you will experience immediately after their ingestion. The sense of well-being is the emotional reason that these substances are addictive. To repeat, in order for these foreign substances to be broken down and excreted, the body must use up its stores of nutrients and energy reserves, thereby reducing your very structure (foundation) and turning it from stone to sand, so to speak. This process is accentuated with the cocaine user. The result is a faster burn out. You may be certain that all other stimulants are doing the same thing to lesser or greater degrees.

Processed foods (nutrient depleted) that have had nutrients taken out to prolong shelf life act on the body in a similar way. When you take in food like bleached flour or refined sugar, what you are eating is the remnant of the original food that has been stripped of vitamins and minerals, and most importantly, enzymes. Because you have not received the vital nutrients these foods should have contained, your hypothalamus (your brain) tells you to eat more. You then crave more sugar or white bread. The body finally succumbs and begins releasing the nutrients from its stores, which are in your liver, bone marrow, gallbladder, etc. Your body pays the price. What you will begin to see is osteoporosis, depression, or fatigue, which are rampant in society today.

Many companies are committed to making the American public aware that these deficiencies are due to inadequate levels of nutrients in the average Americans diet. This is only partially true. The truth is that many people consume a diet that is low in certain vitamins, minerals, and enzymes and yet show no deficiencies in these nutrients. Why is this? I propose that your body has the ability to create all the vitamins, minerals, and enzymes it requires by the power of the mind.

What I propose is that emotions can interfere with proper choices, and lead us to select processed foods, thereby creating abnormal body chemistry. This, in turn, will create a fertile breeding ground for bacteria, viruses, cancer cells, fungus, etc. When our body presents us with symptoms, and we ignore them, it will simply proceed to the next stage. Toxicity, then, is secondary to emotional dis-ease. The fact of the matter is that a healthy individual's daily exposure to toxins is not an issue. There is a study involving patients who were subjected to potential lead poisoning. The patients who were at risk were the ones who already had an insufficient level of calcium in the blood. Logically, we can apply this scenario to other toxicities to which we are all exposed daily.

Before you get too excited and think that this is the ticket to eat like a fool, and still have a positive mental attitude and be healthy, it is not so. This is a huge dilemma or excuse as people look for excuses to postpone changes. With that said I believe that it is more important to have minimal stress in your life than worry about particulars in your diet. The challenge is finding the balance in eating real, wholefoods as a rule, and when faced with toxic or processed foods while traveling or elsewhere trust that your body can handle it.

The purpose of a forest fire: It is a natural aspect of the forest ecology and cycle. Often fire is essential for new growth and germination. The purpose of a volcano: The natural way of cooling off and releasing pressure and can also release alkaline ash into the environment for better soil. The purpose of economic recession is to help with waste reduction; it's a form of a diet for the economy.

In health, there is always a purpose: of gaining weight, a swollen joint, the purpose of the fever to burn off the virus and slow you down (See The Course In Health Workbook on more examples). Having eye problems are associated with not wanting to see what's right in front of you, or the future. Your shoulders relate to what you carry or burdens you bear. If we don't ask what the point is for an illness or condition we will never discover. If we ask the wrong question we will get the wrong answer. The questions we ask with heart illness, cancer, or diabetes is the wrong question because it seeks to answer the external causes.

There are many scientific studies that would support this statement. One particular case study involved multiple personality people who changed from a person with diabetes to a normal within minutes, and back again. The power of the mind is quite unbelievable. So we are now able to grasp that we must look at absorption as well as intake. If your digestion is not functioning optimally due to stress, for instance, you will be unable to absorb nutrients. Have you ever seen a person who eats correctly, yet looks sick? It is the emotional component at work.

WOULDN'T I KNOW IT?

"Doc, this is the way that my entire family has always eaten… everything in moderation. Besides, wouldn't I know it if I had a digestive problem?"

To this point, consider: If cigarettes are harmful to one's health, wouldn't a smoker know it? The answer is yes and no. When a person first begins to smoke, the body protests in the form of coughing, choking, tears, excess saliva production, or any combination thereof. However, if the person ignores these messages, and for a mental/emotional reason decides that he or she is going to continue to smoke, within a few days or weeks, the lungs will literally go into shock and stop giving messages of discomfort. In the same way, is it possible that our digestive systems have stopped giving us messages about some of the foods that we eat? To answer this, we need to look back at our first exposure to solid foods as infants. Leading pediatric nutritionists say that infants are unable to fully digest solid foods until 12 to 18 months of age, when teeth and digestive enzymes have developed. Too many of us are exposed to solid foods as early as 1-3 months of age! The stools of a breastfed baby have an almost sweet smell to them. Contrast this with the distinctly foul odor of the stools of an infant who is fed solid foods early in life. This foul odor indicates that because the foods were incompletely digested in the upper portions of the digestive system, they rotted in the lower small intestine and colon, subsequently releasing toxins into the bloodstream. This is one drastic way in which an infant is forced to communicate with us about the challenges of some of the foods that we feed him. Another way is to spit up food. Yet another is a bloated belly. Rotting, undigested food will cause the little "Buddha" bellies that are considered cute and healthy, when in fact they are the indicator of a baby's digestive distress. Many babies do not exhibit these particular symptoms, yet they are fussy. Fussy babies are trying to tell us something. The pediatrician who explains to the parent that their baby has colic and will "outgrow it" is setting the stage for that baby to ignore his body. Colic is not normal. Just like the smoker's lungs which eventually stop crying out from the noxious stimulus, the infant's digestive system will soon give up and stop producing these messages.

Is it any surprise then, that as adults, we have become numb to the distress signals produced by the digestive system? Many of us cannot discern between foods that nourish our entire bodies, and foods that nourish only our taste buds.

Consider a parable or metaphor of a frog that is placed in a pot of cold water. If this water is heated very gradually, the frog will be unable to sense the slow rise in temperature (Don't think this metaphor is factual; it sounds good). Eventually, without having a clear warning, the frog will succumb to the boiling water and die. Contrast this with putting a frog into a pot of water that is boiling to begin with. Experiencing a clear signal of pain, the frog will immediately jump out to safety. How many of us are like the first frog, contributing to our health challenges via detrimental lifestyle habits whose effects are so subtle and gradual that our bodies are unable to experience a clear signal of danger? Will you agree with me that your body is more complicated than a computer? Or any man-made thing, for that matter. All man-made things have nifty, built-in mechanisms to alert the owner of potential dangers. Should you expect less from your body? It has the same built-in communication system, but our penchant for control and independence has muffled our ability to be in tune with these signals. We use drugs, pills, addictions, etc. to turn off the signal. Another thought to ponder is that most of us have been taught to ignore symptoms from an age that we don't even have a memory of.

So, what determines your current level of health? (See workbook exercise 1). Most physicians are inclined to believe that our health is the result of our genetics and a combination of luck, as well as the choices we make.

Put yourself in my place, as you hear a patient explaining to me, "Doc, I just can't believe that drinking coffee could have anything to do with my aching joints. Tons of people drink way more than I do, and they don't have this problem." Or. "Everyone has stress! How could stress be causing my high blood pressure when others have stress and are fine?"

Your genetics and the specific weak links (and strong ones) that come with them are affected by your lifestyle habits. Your weak link may be your skin. Your neighbor's maybe his heart. For others, it may be a respiratory challenge, trouble with weight, heartburn, constipation and/or diarrhea, chronic cough, sinus pain, an intestinal disorder, autoimmune disorder, etc. Regardless of your genetic predispositions, you can choose to live in a way that minimizes your chances of having to deal with them. If you can sincerely rule out genetics when you approach your personal health issues, you are approaching your conditions with an attitude which can facilitate real healing. Embrace your weak links as lessons, which you have manifested on this physical journey of yours. I am not trying to tell you that you did not inherit DNA from your parents. I am encouraging you to look at the reasons you may have manifested these specific genes and not others.

We must always ask, "Where does the power lie once I have taken responsibility for everything in my life?" Blaming the stock market, your ex, your children, whatever it is, is always easier than accepting responsibility for yourself. But it is also giving your power away, time and again, sometimes to family, sometimes to total strangers.

In my practice I find this to be incredibly consistent. Patients come to see me wanting reassurance that they are okay, that they are not to blame, and all they have to do is take this pill, or go through this procedure and they can continue to live as they have always lived. The reality is you brought this condition into your life. I can't do a thing for you to heal your body. I can do magic in the sense that I can give pills and treatments to "make the pain go away." The truth is that curing is of the body, and healing is of the mind. Curing of the physical body is temporary and belongs within our concept of time. Healing is of the mind. It transcends time and the physical and brings us to new levels. Healing can be accomplished only one way—by you. No one can do it for you.

Let's look at would-be exceptions to this paradigm, such as an inherited genetic illness. First, ask yourself why "genetic" conditions are on the rise. I recently read in a medical journal that doctors have linked ear infections to genetics. This is another example of the medical system telling people what they want to hear. The general public wants to hear that it is not their fault, they could not have prevented this, or it's just bad luck. Several years ago I attended a planning session for a multi-million dollar "spiritual retreat center." The investors, natural therapists, and the business advisors were brainstorming. The MBA advisor gave his input as to the financial prospects of the venture. Simply stated, he informed the group "You have to find out what the public wants, and then give it to them." I would like to propose a different thought structure. If Jesus were to operate through this philosophy, do you think he would have bothered with the Sermon on the Mount? Would he continue to tell his trusting audience that their healing occurs because of their faith? Imagine if you can, Jesus telling a mother that her child's blindness is genetic, and would she please take him home and deal with it. Or would he start a fundraising program to generate millions of dollars to begin research for a cure? And surely, since he already had the attention of his audience, he could convince them that he alone could treat these ills with drugs, and threaten anyone else who tried to treat with drugs with a lawsuit for "practicing medicine without a license."

Again, Marianne Williamson talks about how powerful we truly are. "It is our light, not our darkness, that most frighten us... Our deepest fear is not that we are inadequate. Our deepest fear is that we are powerful beyond measure."

Your power lies within you. You always have the choice to manifest your present condition, health or otherwise. Or you can spend your time and energy selecting your scapegoats externally, thereby giving up your power. Our natural and mainstream medical systems teach us the opposite.

The disease first becomes possible when we deviate from homeostasis, not genetics, bad luck or chance. When your choices in your daily lives expose you to toxins, excesses, deficiencies, stressful thoughts, or not understanding our feelings, we ultimately get sick. Remember: The Earth is not the center of the universe.

Toxins include those chemicals that we consume through food, water and air (pesticides, refined sugar, carbon monoxide) and those that are produced within our own digestive tracts due to rotting and undigested foods. These toxins are chemically akin to the toxins used to embalm cadavers. Note that illness first becomes possible, not inevitable, with exposure to these toxins. Excess meaning: too much caffeine, refined sugar, processed food, sleep, alcohol, shopping, stress, etc.

Deficiency meaning: lack of nutrients in our food from farming practices, processing, or lack of consumption. Deficiency also includes touch, love, and fun.

Emotional factors that contribute to our illness include job dissatisfaction, unresolved emotional hurts, etc. Make no mistake about it; our lifestyle habits determine how susceptible or resistant we are to illness. Do ants infest a spotless kitchen floor, eventually coaxing the cook to spill food or do ants seek out and thrive on the floor that is abundant with spilled food? With the same understanding, you can see that blaming the bug that is going around for your sniffles is an incomplete way of thinking. Is your body the appropriate soil for toxins to take root? Listen to some of the explanations I hear: "Doc, it's not a toxin that caused my sore throat. They took a culture and found strep. That's why I'm taking these antibiotics."

Well, guess what? Streptococcus bacteria naturally live within our upper respiratory tract. It is only when the balance is upset that changes occur. We must understand that bacteria are opportunistic; they flourish when they have the appropriate soil to do so. Could it be that your indulgence in ice cream (refined sugar) combined with excessive stress at work lately and lack of restful sleep due to worry were the root causes of your susceptibility to strep throat?

What kind of an impact do you suppose that underlying toxicity and associated weakening of one's defenses have on how well one endures or recovers from illness caused by non-toxic factors? Lifestyle habits that support low toxicity and strong defenses will most certainly allow the body to use every last ounce of its potential to endure any challenges and maintain or restore health.

The power of the mind to rise above deficiencies is a reality, for some deficiencies do not manifest as conditions. The mind is a powerful thing.

TO SUMMARIZE THE CAUSE OF ILLNESS

If we know the cause of illness we can therefore claim how to heal illness. Mainstream medical research and science have shown the cause of most illness to be due to nutritional factors and stress. A past Surgeon General estimates that 68 percent of all deaths in the United States are directly related to dietary factors. So why is it that we cannot reverse these conditions after taking out the nutritional culprit? The answer to this question goes deeper in analyzing the previous question. To know the cause is to know the cure. We know with certainty that refined sugar causes illness by weakening the immune system, among many other negative health effects. We know with certainty that hydrogenated oils and bleached flour cause heart disease. The broader question would be: Why do some people choose these foods over others? Mental-emotional blocks: anger, fear, guilt, insecurity, etc., lead us to behaviors or choices that are not health promoting.

I believe it is not helpful for a doctor to merely put patients on a diet (i.e. telling patients that sugar is bad, white flour is bad, etc.). This doctor's orders makes the situation worse! The reason being is that most people inherently know that processed foods and refined sugar are not health promoting. Most people know that insufficient sleep, excess alcohol, tobacco, etc., are not health promoting. When a doctor tells someone to stop a behavior that is not health promoting without addressing the reason why this person has chosen these destructive foods, it only adds stress.

Why do some people drink excess caffeine, eat in excess, and not sleep enough? The simple reason: stress and a way to cope. So if the doctor tells the patient to stop the coping mechanism without addressing the stressor, the doctor is making the situation worse.

How this works is a little complicated, but when understood makes a lot of sense. When an obese patient comes to see me they often ask "Doctor, can you put me on a diet? You put Jennifer on one because she lost a lot of weight." I reply that I never put people on a diet. Within the word diet is the word "die" and most people would rather die than do it. People are not inherently bad or lazy; there is always a reason why someone becomes overweight. Many don't ask the correct question: Why am I overweight? The reason why many don't ask is that it is too painful to ask. In all the obesity cases I have seen, all patients have had some emotional trauma, usually centered on sexuality. The weight that is put on is a goal-oriented, biological process. The goal (subconscious) is to put weight on their body to create a buffer between them and what they fear. The weight sometimes may give them a sense of power or control. Regardless, it is intended and purposeful.

If a doctor had a magic wand that could remove excess weight and bring a patient to their ideal weight it would be dangerous because emotionally the person would most likely not have the ability to cope. If you watch dieters or reality television weight loss shows we see that the bigger challenge is keeping the weight off as opposed to losing the weight. Unless the person addresses the subconsciously purposeful reason for getting obese, they will return to that pattern.

When a doctor or dietitian tells their patient not to eat certain foods (i.e. donuts, potato chips, etc.) because they are making them fat, but instead eat broccoli, the patient is being told that something that tastes good to them (donuts) is bad and something that taste bad (broccoli) is good. Because at the moment they believe that weight loss will bring them happiness they are on board and they dedicate themselves to the diet. They eat the broccoli and eliminate the donuts with sheer willpower. They start to lose weight but soon their emotions, thoughts, and beliefs start to enter. Unresolved issues that initially drove this person to donuts for comfort pop up. They see the donut and they begin to rationalize that one donut is okay. I have been so good. I can cheat this one time. They eat the donut and it tastes great! They now go back and associate pleasure with the donut, and pain with the healthy broccoli. They consciously and subconsciously feel guilt or shame or failure. Because these negative feelings hurt they begin to deny that they really *want* or *need* to lose weight. The entire diet becomes a negative association. Doctor has done harm. Now let's look at a physics approach to change. I ask the patient why they want to lose weight; I have them clarify their values and look at their purpose in life. We address the emotional trauma or conflict that may have contributed to the weight issue. The patient understands that the process to heal is going to create a change or disturbance in their status quo. I ask them if they are ready to rock the boat. If they are not, we don't proceed. If they say yes, something needs to change. I then explain that I will not provide them a diet. I will teach them the difference between foods that heal and foods that push them further away from their values and purpose. I also explain that the foods we choose or don't choose are rooted in emotions and past conflict. I recommend some foods, food combinations, food supplements, exercise that suits them, and further explain to them that they are free to take these recommendations and apply them to their life. I give them some rules to follow when eating healthy and toxic food. In the process of eating the patient tells themselves without prejudice what the food is going to do to them. This broccoli is moving me closer to health, and ultimately closer to my values and purpose. This donut is moving me closer to obesity, arthritis, and diabetes, and further away from my values and purpose. I am good person for wanting to change, my honesty about the donut is helpful, and at this time it is more important to me to satisfy my physical and emotional taste buds, than it is to heal. The most important part of this dialogue and process is to be truly gentle and optimistic towards yourself. No judgment.

When this process is done correctly—while the patient is addressing the emotional wounds that have led them to donuts and other soothing foods—they become aware of the emotional connection between their diet and mind. They allow themselves to be human and take the wrong road. In doing so something connects internally and the person with their own drive stands up and says this donut tastes awful.

Remember the seat of the taste bud is in the mind and not on the tongue: a fact that requires a full understanding to embrace change and process addictions. One other dialogue I use with people is hypothetically offering them crack cocaine or heroin. Without exception the person I make the offer to aggressively declines. I ask them why? I have the best stuff. They respond to me that they are turned off by the offer. I persist and explain that it will blow their mind and it will feel good. They maintain their disgust and explain that they associate pain with heroin or crack cocaine because of what it could do to their relationships, job, or possible incarceration. I then become the devil's advocate and explain that many people associate great pleasure with these drugs, and if I offered it to a person using these drugs they would do anything to access them. We then go on to discuss that many people associate the same disgust or pain with unhealthy foods. The conversation ends and hopefully this person can develop a love for themselves that creates healthy food choices.

The same applies to exercise. The number of studies that show how exercise is beneficial to health is astronomical. The same amount of studies shows how exercise is critical for cancer patients, diabetics, and most other health issues. The same question applies: Why are people not exercising? The complicated reason is that of a lack of love for themselves. A person who loves themselves is active, eats well, and takes care of their body, finances, and relationships. The simple answer is it requires change, values clarification and addressing the self-sabotage issues that have led the person to be sedentary.

The foods that you crave and the foods you are allergic to all have a deeper meaning. The harmful foods you crave that produce ill health have the potential to be the failure that brings success. It is no different than using harmful foods to give you cues to your emotional issues to bring you to resolve.

CHANGE OVERVIEW

The "how and why" change occurs is tied to purpose and virtues. When we have a powerful *why* the *how* comes easy. Our inspiration is intrinsic. This allows us to act "response" "able" and be willing to endure pain and pleasure in the pursuit of our purpose. We generally move in one of two directions: Towards pleasure and purpose, or away from pain. Our healthcare system is solely based on moving away from pain. I propose that healing only occurs when we move toward pleasure and purpose. Without a radical change in addressing health as a whole, we will continue to see illness rates and addictions increase.

Health is not just what we eat, or how much we exercise or the genes passed down from our parents. Think for a moment how financial stress can affect your physical health. Just look at the top five reasons people go bankrupt. The number one reason is medical expenses. Even in countries such as Canada that have government health plans, medical costs are a leading cause of bankruptcy. It is well-established that financial problems cause medical problems. You may ask if this is a chicken or egg question... do the health problems cause the financial illness or does the financial illness manifest into health problems. In a recent study, researchers found an absolute connection with low credit scores correlating to poor health. What this is saying is if you have poor credit it is very likely due to the lack of self-control surrounding money. This, in turn, manifests to lack of self-control in your health. An examination of people with poor credit reveals overspending being the common denominator. This action is an internal decision that is directly linked to self-control; the majority of those with poor credit will blame their overspending on external factors: luck, chance or genetics. Overspending is a self-control virtue connected with the self-control that drives health issues.

When a person has illness in their finances, relationships and/or physical health there is an action, addiction, crutch, or something that makes them stuck.

The first hurdle is finding what the action, addiction, or crutch is. The second hurdle is changing the action or behavior. Sounds simple—because it is. Let's look into the addictions that bring people to illness.

We can first look at finances. Why do people have financial problems? Generally, they spend more than they make and they don't save money.

The deeper question is *why* do they spend more than they make? The answer to this is connected with how to change. Our overspending is linked to addiction. Changing oneself is overcoming the addiction. This book will help guide us through the process. Many people will be raising their hands claiming that their money problems stem from their divorce, medical bills, unexpected expenses or job loss.

I work with many financially successful people and as you would expect each one strongly believes and defends that their finances are not related to luck, chance or genetics but how they approach money, like discipline or hard work along with other traits related to money and efficacy... like virtues.

Hang tight as the connection with relationships, your physical health and money will become all too obvious as you read this book. To understand health and healing we must first understand cause and effect. Disease is a goal-orientated biological process.

Let's go through the intellectual process of change, and take the mystery out of addiction and illness.

1st - Health is not external.

2nd - Discover the addiction.

3rd - Discovering medical and natural treatments that are ineffective.

4th - Uncovering the scientific myth.

5th - Understanding principles of health and healing.

6th - Taking action steps to affect change*. (See The Course In Health Workbook)

Change meaning changing a part of you that no longer serves your Grand Purpose. We see these changes when someone overcomes any addiction. When someone who in the past made bad choices by stealing or being indulgent with food or drugs truly changes, they will be confronted with a situation in which they can choose the old path or rise above. In these situations when the person is tempted to steal, their consciousness tells them that the old me would have chosen the painful path. "The new me" doesn't choose that path. The choice is easy because they have truly changed. How one changes is the question I asked myself for years. The answer is simple and may not require the above six steps. Simply deciding that the new you chooses life and love.

DOCTOR SAND VS. DOCTOR ROCK
External vs. Internal

Telling patients it is luck, chance or genetics makes the patient weak, not accountable. Treatments assume the patient cannot heal on their own. Teaching patients the cause helps the patient become whole.

-Doctor Sand scenario goes like this: Doctor explains that the ear infection (otitis media) is a serious condition that could cause SERIOUS hearing loss, and is VERY painful, further explaining that the condition is caused by a virus, and we don't know what caused the problem. I recommend we wait and see if it resolves on its own.

-Mother Fear: Deaf?! Pain?! What can we do about it?

-Doctor Sand: I meant to say... antibiotics or tubes in the ear.

-Doctor Rock scenario goes like this: Doctor Rock explains that your child has an inflamed middle ear. It is a virus, similar to the common cold. The child's immune system is somehow weakened and needs to be strengthened. Dr. Rock further explains the other component is emotional or stress factors. Doctor Rock explains that almost all children with ear infections do not want to hear what's going around them, often parents fighting.

-Mother Calm: Doctor, how does the immune system weaken?

-Doctor Rock explains that the bug (virus) is of little significance if the internal environment is in order. Just like your hot tub or fish tank when you check the pH balance and keep it clean, viruses do not make a home in your hot tub. If you allow the balance to go too far off, the virus has a place to live.

-Dr. Rock asks parent: Does the mosquito create the swamp or does the swamp attract the mosquito? If the hot tub goes off balance it becomes a swamp, the mosquito flies by and realizes he has a great place to live and breed. But, when the mosquito flies by the hot tub that is cared for it stays away and it can't thrive there. The virus, parasite, fungus or bacteria are no different. They all need certain conditions to live and grow. If you take away their food they go away. Homeostasis/balance is determined by many things including hydration, macro and micronutrients, sleep, electromagnetic stress, exercise, and other stressors. If you don't change the swamp back to clean water the virus will stay. Why do you think that out of the hundreds of times you have been exposed to a virus (or any bug) you have not caught the virus. Simply put, your body was not a suitable environment for the bug.

-Doctor Rock may ask Parent Calm how much refined sugar or processed food the child is eating, or if he is exercising, etc.

-Doctor Rock reassures Parent Calm that this virus will run its course and that there was a purpose in its existence.

-Mother Calm is now Mother Empowered. Mother Empowered's light comes on. She explains to the doctor that she can see how illness is a biological process and has a purpose. She recounts to Doctor Rock that yes things have been stressful at home with a lot of arguing between parents, things are rushed and child is eating a lot of processed food and watching a lot of television. Mother goes on to explain that if this amazing virus did not come along it wouldn't have made us slow down and look at the stresses. Mother Empowered becomes Mother Thankful and Mother Responsible.

Note that Doctor Sand's visit was very quick and efficient; Doctor Rock's office visit was a lot longer and comprehensive.

Doctor Sand versus Doctor Rock's office visit is about a parent being open to change versus a parent being closed to change.

I have the utmost respect for well-intentioned physicians. Our medical system's pursuit of 'cures' is what has brought us back to responsible health. If we hadn't spent trillions of dollars trying to find a cure for cancer, arthritis, or diabetes, we might be still thinking that all we need is more money. If we had not spent the last forty years having some of the most intelligent people researching cures, we would just think we need more time. Most important to note is that the medical system is patient-directed. What you ask for is what you receive.

A PEACE OF CHANGE

Of the drugs that are available today that will remain in circulation despite their proven toxicity are those that give pain relief. It is incredible to understand the psychology behind people's choices of moving away from pain at any extent. If asked if the pain is good or bad, most would claim it is bad. The reality is pain is a blessing; it tells us what we are doing is in error. If we didn't experience pain, there would be a disaster. Consider the simple scenario of touching the hot stove. The immediate pain warns of the damage the heat will do to our skin. When it comes to pain it is essential to see the cause and effect of pain with your relationships. If you don't treat your partner with respect, you feel the pain of being alone. If you don't respect the principles of living within your means, you experience many financial pains from high-interest credit cards, bank fees, etc.

There are several problems with the modern medical model. The first is that its entire existence is based on external cause and external cure, and second, all treatment is combative. The law of physics will refute the solution. Every action has an equal and opposite reaction! This is Newton's third law in physics. When we fight back the physics law will still apply even if we have justified it.

To look into the law of physics, we can see that there are two ways to get results. The first is the nonviolent way: like the principles of Gandhi or Martin Luther King or Jesus. The second is violent opposition—war (i.e., the war on cancer, or any war). The law of physics causes the second way to abort itself. The force that is applied in these areas is countered with an equal opposition. Dropping a bowling ball on the ground causes a force onto the ground. What is difficult to observe is that the ground responds with an opposite and equal force. If you punch the wall, it is both your force and the force of the wall pushing back that causes pain. When force is used there is resistance. When a war is over, the result is turmoil, conflict, and resentment.

For example, if I wanted you to come up on stage at a lecture I was giving I could do one of two things. The first option would be to come up to you in your seat and start tugging on your arm, forcing or dragging you up on stage. As I pulled harder, you would resist to that same degree. The second way to get you on stage would be to walk up to you, put my arm on your shoulder, reassure you that I wouldn't do anything to hurt or embarrass you and gently walk with you to the stage.

Which scenario do you think would provide me with a more relaxed (happy) subject? I think it is obvious that getting someone on stage is not the challenge. The challenge is to have a person who is more relaxed. Parallel this with getting rid of the breast cancer you have been diagnosed with. Yes, cutting off your breast does get rid of cancer at the location. But, what are the reactions that physics will have? Wouldn't *embracing* the breast cancer (as I did with the subject for my demonstration) in a loving way be more productive?

A while back our family purchased a puppy. With this comes the responsibility of training this new member of our family. I was introduced to a technique in training that incorporates all of the non-violent approaches that I am discussing. This dog training technique involves NEVER using force—the thing that most people use to train their pets or children even. The person who was explaining this technique explained that whenever you use a force on a pet the animal will resist with an equal force. For those who might be thinking, yeah but it works... think again. The animal will be submissive to you because of your greater force; however, given the opportunity, they will rebel. They may turn on the owner or a child or act badly when force is not present. Just like a prisoner, they will submit to the force of being restrained, however, given the opportunity, they will rebel. Going back to the dog training, what you see with animals trained in this manner is amazing. A dog will submit and obey just as well and most often better than when combative tools are used. I must also say that applying these techniques takes more time, energy and patience in the early stages, but they ultimately pay off.

John Lions, a famous horse trainer, advocates the same philosophy. I would choose an animal or friend that was trained in nonviolent areas over violent ways. Just as the movements of Gandhi, Martin Luther King, and Jesus—we see no force. And the results are lasting. A crucial distinction is that the non-violent approach does take courage, patience, trust, clarity, faith, etc. If these values are not exercised, then the ego will manipulate the mind with fear and prejudice, going back to the need to use external forces.

These same principles apply to health, both emotional and physical. What we are seeing is that our current medical system is proving its lack of worth by its lack of success. The medical model is one of the newest forms of treatment (less than 200 years old).

Natural therapies have survived so many years because of the fact they are helpful at improving symptoms and the action of the treatment is not harmful. Acupuncture, spinal adjustments, homeopathic, and herbal remedies were used 3000 years ago. These therapies work *with* the human body, not against it. The difference can be seen when we take a look at the terminology: Allopathic (medical) and homeopathy. The word "allo" means against; "homeo" means with.

At this point you may be hesitant because your experience with acupuncture, chiropractic or other natural treatments was unsuccessful. This is a serious question that both natural and modern medical therapies face. Is the treatment proven and, more importantly, effective?

Let's look at the herbs, acupuncture points, spinal manipulations, etc., that were used 3000 years ago. They are basically identical to those used today. If these techniques were harmful or did not produce results, 3000 years of clinical results and research would have deemed these techniques or treatments to be harmful or ineffective. Almost all are proven nontoxic, or have low side effects. The question that remains: Are these natural treatments ineffective as tools for healing or just relief care? These natural approaches comply with the Hippocratic Oath.

First: do no harm. Second: produce results. The question then remains why they do not correct 100 percent of cases. Or do they address the root cause or only superficial symptoms by giving relief and kicking the can down the road?

If we insist on framing our health within that incomplete external paradigm, we will come up against the same wall of physics and the law of force. The force is gentler on the body with natural therapy, to be sure, but it will still elicit an equal and opposite reaction, which will hopefully equate to a cure. But does it heal? No. Healing does not exist within the modern incomplete paradigm in which we work. The point is that natural therapy is definitely the more logical of choices for suppressing some symptoms. The mainstream modern medical excels at suppressing other symptoms. But natural therapy is no different than the current medical approach, which hinders the patient's growth in the great majority of cases.

When looking for medical help whether it is a supplement, drug or any treatment, it is essential to look at the cumulative effect of taking action.

To think that just a supplement or drug can fix a problem alone is not realistic. Looking at a vegetable garden is helpful. If some of what you planted were not growing, you would need to look at the nutrients in the soil and possibly supplement the soil. You would also look at sunlight, water, temperature, structural aspects of the plants and tender loving care. Often it is a cumulative effect. One plus one can equal three or four. Taking away something toxic to an illness is not magic.

In health it is the same; without addressing the underlying stress or emotional factor, the pill will not have a positive effect. Sometimes it is exercising, breathing, stretching, talking, or a combination, that will get the results. The missing piece in most medical practices is the action required alongside the pill or treatment which includes the exercise; whether the exercise is physical exercise or mental exercise.

"The spirit in which an act is conducted is more powerful than the act itself"(Unknown). This will cross over into the placebo effect in the chapters to come. When the spirit is to fight an illness with external means we are doomed for failure. This also applies to the war on terrorism or the war on drugs. It does not matter if the approach is medical or natural. I have studied many who have had spontaneous remission from cancer, from my own clinical experience to the work of Norman Cousins, to recent scientific research. In these remissions some do so alongside taking chemo or radiation, some changing their diet or taking natural remedies, among other ways. The underlying foundation of the remission is what is addressed in this book. To be considered spontaneous remission no treatment (radiation or natural) should be considered connected to the remission.

In a well-conducted study titled *The natural history of invasive breast cancers detected by screening mammography*, it concluded that up to 22 percent of all screened breast cancer diagnosis underwent spontaneous remission(Arch Intern Med. 2008 Nov 24). Profound to me is the 80/20 rule in finances, relationships and health.

Whereas it is repeated throughout the remarkable pattern of only 20 percent of the public having saved adequately for retirement, only 20 percent of relationships/marriage that are healthy functioning, with no codependency, no divorce, no infidelity, etc. With health we see only 20 percent not on medications having the ability to heal. I believe this 20 percent can easily shift to 80 percent if the internal principles are applied.

I believe what has allowed for the healing of these "cancer" growths is the spirit in which the diagnosis was handled. Those who heal share one common trait: working with, learning from, or embracing their condition, whether it is cancer, heart disease, headaches or a skin condition. Furthermore, not blaming and not being embarrassed or ashamed of their manifestation. Another requirement for healing is having a purpose in life, or being "on purpose."

In the pursuit of health, most people are given drugs, vitamins, surgery, or other treatments. The fact that a lot of these therapies excel at masking symptoms, the conclusion people make is that they have arrived at their destination and their map is reinforced as being correct. The vitamin fixed me! Conditioning starts here.

The light on your dashboard comes on (symptom) warning that your brakes need repair. Putting a black piece of tape over the dash light or disconnecting the light makes the symptom go away. Would you pay for that type of service? Our paradigm for our automobile mechanic is consistent with getting to the root of the problem. We are all aware that ignoring the brake problem will not fix it. We know that it will turn a simple brake pad job into a complicated, expensive rotor and caliber job. Even if we don't have the time or money to fix the brakes, our paradigm on auto mechanics tells us that we need to respect the repair and get it done correctly. In conclusion, we do not get rewarded for ignoring the brake light. We are conditioned to having our cars repaired correctly.

The map we currently use for health is built on sand; I would like you to build your health foundation on solid rock.

You may think that asking well-intentioned educated medical doctors, naturopaths, dentists and chiropractors for assistance is good enough. You may settle for answers from these doctors who tell you to keep on searching using the wrong map and all that you need is more time, a better insurance plan or more money. Or, that it is normal what you are experiencing. Where does this settling leave you? Is our health getting better or worse? Are we spending more time, money and energy in attaining health?

It is a concern that your medical provider is not taught the difference between healthcare and disease care. The well-intentioned professional sells you "disease care" disguised as healthcare. Is your doctor forthcoming in explaining that the pill or treatment that he gives you does not cure the condition? Is this consistent with the original Hippocratic Oath?

If you can remember the 1970s, one of the leading advertisers in mainstream medical journals was cigarette manufacturers. The mainstream medical journals accepted smoking advertising and generated lots of money from it. At present, our doctors and medical journals do not allow such advertising and educate against smoking. When doctors supported tobacco and told people it was okay to smoke in the 1970s, did that mean tobacco was okay?

Are the recommended vitamins, vaccines, pharmaceutical drugs, etc. the "new" tobacco that well-intentioned doctors are supporting?

Is the quality of our lives worse off than ever? We see illness rates increase at alarming rates. Our medical systems (modern and natural) are failing. Do not confuse quality of life with quantity of life. If our medical system excels at keeping people alive, are they improving people's quality of life? Is there a difference between illness care and healthcare?

If you were looking for financial health, would you rather have an extensive line of credit or a source of income that provides you with continual income? The large line of credit may give an illusion that you have money and take away the symptoms, but in time it will fall like a house of cards. Disease care is like borrowing money; healthcare is like making wise investments.

I like to use financial analogies with health because of the remarkable similarity. People and businesses who uphold a complete paradigm on finances consistently enjoy healthy business or financial ease. I have personally found those financially in control (self-control... not necessarily rich) are easier to work with and consistently access higher levels of health than those with financial illness (i.e. bad credit).

The same can be said about insurance. It is called health insurance but should be called illness insurance. We call flood insurance correctly.

Ironically our medical system feeds off the opposite attributes of the complete paradigm of health. It encourages and rewards people to not take responsibility. Our financial system does the opposite. Banks and credit institutions only reward the healthy. Banks and creditors add fees or charge higher interest rates for bad credit. They offer rewards and better interest rates for the financially healthy. It makes perfect sense.

The interesting point here is that healthcare does not sell; what sells is negative emotions like fear, scarcity or magical thinking. Our medical system sells disease care by fear or by the magic bullet. Disease care is sold like the unattainable lottery ticket. Watch the lottery ticket commercial, not much different from the pharma ad.

I have looked hard at my approach to health (relationship, physical and financial). Many do not want to hear what I am saying because it is too painful and contrary to their approach in rationalizing their behavior. Those who are truly successful in these areas do not need to hear it because they are already living the paradigm and take responsibility for their lives.

It is interesting that many religious leaders sway people to feel better about themselves versus calling people out to change. Doctors do the same thing—telling patients that their condition is not their fault. Our society is partly changing in the right direction with lecturers and educators telling things how they are; telling people what they need to hear versus what they want to hear.

The experience I have had in over 20 years in medicine is that all conditions have an emotional component. Our medical system doesn't even scratch the surface. My practice has been directed to addressing the root of the patient's health issue. Discussing emotions, feelings and the stress management side of a condition is challenging and time-consuming. I have taken the opposite approach to selling healthcare.

The same way an evangelist or salesperson persuades someone to buy into their "deal," our healthcare system is no different. The medical system is a business—successful at selling their products. Most people do not think about medicine and being "sold." The fact is that the sales approach has been mastered and perfected. In many cases it uses the best (I consider the worst) tactic to sell: It's called fear.

The efforts and techniques used by the natural and the modern medical system are used to convert your beliefs about medicine into a religion.

The important thing is to distinguish between the religious component of healthcare and the spiritual aspect of healing. Having a belief in the healing process is crucial to healing. Putting your acupuncturist, medical doctor, or chiropractor on a pedestal and unknowingly worshiping them, their practice or the pills they prescribe moves you further away from true healing.

We believe that our health must be bought or insured. Or that the secret to our health is in drugs, vitamins, new treatments, or having access to the right doctors. This belief has been carved into many people's minds. This belief is not backed by fact or logic. There is a positive relationship between money and better health. At the same time, those who consume more drugs or hold better insurance plans do not have better health. The facts show that Americans consume the most pharmaceuticals, and pay the most per capita on health yet they lag far beyond the rest of the industrialized world in overall health and longevity.

How does the medical system brainwash people? It does by using high-pressure sales techniques that don't come across as high pressure but rather as a sincere concern for you. These high-pressure techniques include using shame and guilt when we question or oppose the god-like doctor or the practices and beliefs of these doctors. The high-pressure sales techniques mislead by abusing science to sell their treatment. Mainstream medical and natural medicine are equally to blame for the misuse of the word scientific.

What is the difference between being brainwashed and having an incorrect belief? Take a step back without skepticism and ask yourself, what if I was brainwashed? How would you know? When we watch children in the Middle East brainwashed by these same techniques on anti-American doctrine we are amazed. We see these innocent children chant "kill the Americans" or "kill the Jews." If we ask these people if they are brainwashed, they would deny it. How would they know it? It is a very difficult pattern to break. How do you un-brainwash the anti-American sentiment and terrorists in the Middle East? The answer is simple and the process is difficult. The answer lies in education and having people be accountable. This process requires people realizing that over time their beliefs and actions are not bringing them closer to their goals. In time they will challenge their paradigm and beliefs on war and choose a different path.

Is it safe to say that those teaching the brainwashing are brainwashed? Whether it is terrorists or medical educators, both are equally sincere in their beliefs. If brainwashing is too harsh a word, look back to those holding onto the notion that the world was the center of the universe to protect their belief of biblical teachings.

Medical students are taught one way and don't have the option to do things differently. They must conform to the strict protocols. The process of Residency is the AMA's method of getting new doctors to conform to their misleading and controlling approach to healthcare.

When it comes to the medical student there is one more twist. They have many years and over $200,000 dollars invested in this belief system. This type of investment is different from a house that is over $200,000 underwater that you can walk away from. The years invested in a medical degree with student loans that don't go away force people to stay in the profession and conform. As previously quoted, *"It is difficult to get a man to understand something, when his salary depends on his not understanding it."* (Upton Sinclair)

Our mainstream media's salary depends on the advertisers that control them. Our medical mainstream wage depends on drug companies and insurance companies that control them. Our political/ legal system is dependent on the lobbyists that control them.

At this point can we agree that health comes from within the patient and not from the doctor, the treatment or the pill?

Unfortunately the medical business model uses doctors, and in turn, they profit by prescribing drugs, vitamins, and treatments, then, get people hooked on the system. Once you start on drugs (recreational or prescription) it is a slippery slope. Big pharma are the dealers, the ones marketing and pushing the drugs. Our nation is becoming addicted to drugs, first because they are asking for an easy way out, and second, because doctors are willing to enable and profit from it. There is little difference in the beliefs that are held by street drug dealers, and prescription drug dealers. Those dealing drugs use rationalization or compartmentalization to enable their service: "If I don't deal the drugs someone else will."

About 90 percent of drugs only help 30-50 percent of the people. Analysis of this stat is alarming. If we applied this to finances, we would go broke fast.

The British Medical Journal's "Clinical Evidence" analyzed medical treatments to evaluate which are supported by sufficient reliable evidence (BMJ, 2007). They reviewed approximately 2,500 treatments and found:

- 13 percent were found to be beneficial
- 23 percent were likely to be beneficial
- Eight percent were as likely to be harmful as beneficial
- Six percent were unlikely to be beneficial
- Four percent were likely to be harmful or ineffective
- 46 percent were unknown whether they were efficacious or harmful

In the late 1970s, the US government conducted a similar evaluation and found a strikingly similar result. They found that only 10 to 20 percent of medical treatment had evidence of efficacy (Office of Technology Assessment, 1978).

SECTION 6

ADDICTIONS ARE HIDDEN IN ALL CONDITIONS

Consumers are conditioned to believe that addiction is a disease. Approximately 50 years ago people addicted to drugs or alcohol were considered morally flawed, lacked discipline, and were self-centered, among other character flaws. By giving people the label of disease by calling them sick, they were not considered bad. What a relief! What we have seen is this disease model shifting one addiction to another. The person addicted to alcohol stops and becomes addicted to cigarettes, food or something else.

- A gullible person does not believe they are gullible.
- An alcoholic does not believe their drinking is a problem.
- Your eyes project outwards and do not see yourself.
- Most addictions are not admitted to or seen by the afflicted.

We all eat. How do you know your addiction is not food? Fasting is the fastest way to determine. You can be addicted to any aspect of food: carbohydrates, fats, processed foods, sugar. You can also be addicted to excess calories. I propose that all illness is linked to that individual's addiction and vice, with no exception.

Incredibly, the symptoms of abstaining from food (during a fast) are identical to the symptoms a person addicted to alcohol or drugs displays when abstaining or detoxing. Remarkably many people go through the stage of recovery by abstaining from any addicted substance and succeed in the initial stage, usually lasting the first three to five days, then later succumb to the vice.

The categories of addictions include 1) Substance 2) Impulse Control 3) Behavioral.

- **Substance Addictions:** Alcohol, Food, Tobacco, Recreational Drug, Pharma Drug.
- **Impulse Control:** Gambling, stealing, starting fires, acts of anger or violence.
- **Behavioral:** Food, sex, computers/phone/internet/social media, exercise, porn, shopping, seeking pain, working, playing video games, sun tanning, self-help books.

Other under-the-radar addictions are linked to certain behaviors that receive secondary gains like perfectionism, unrelenting standards, being good, right, or perfect, power, money accumulation, drama, conflict, worry.

Believing the unsupported science that addiction is gene-based is problematic. The accepting of the disease model is in denial of facts. Specifically, what triggered the person to use drugs, alcohol or other substances obsessively? Breaking it down into psychological triggers or psychological symptoms shows it is the same as other compulsive behaviors like shopping, exercising, working or cleaning. Addiction is essentially a compulsive issue or a way to deal with pain or conflict. If the person has been taught that the addictive substance is the way to deal with pain or stress there should be no surprise in the addiction.

The symptoms associated with drugs, alcohol, shopping, exercising, or working addictions are many. They often translate to medical symptoms, yet the root of the problem is a social or psychological problem. Our natural and modern doctors are pushing their customers to take pills or treatments to deal with their stress and pain.

Drug companies make money by getting people addicted and make money getting people off drugs, with drugs. The pharmaceutical industry has grown to control much of what is taught to doctors. It is a freight train that is difficult to stop. People in pharmaceutical sales who have no certification as medical professionals are paid well to sell drugs to medical professionals. Have you ever taken a course on marketing or sales? I find it disturbing and troubling because of the lack of virtue to get the sale.

Pharmaceutical companies have a legal path to drug distribution through doctors and pharmacies. A few years ago pharmaceutical companies attempted to increase their drug dealer force by seeking chiropractic physicians with the ability to dispense pain meds (seeing that chiropractic physicians are one of the gatekeepers of people with back pain). Thankfully the chiropractic profession declined the seduction. The point is that the drug company's clear objective is to get people on drugs. Nabisco wants you addicted to Oreo cookies and adds chemicals that make it nearly impossible to have only one. Cigarette companies put chemicals in that increase demand.

Why do 87 percent of people over 65 years old take medication? Recent studies showed 70 percent of Americans are on at least one prescription. Fair to say that many of these people are or are becoming addicted to these meds... nobody talks about it... the dilemma big pharma has is its desire to get people hooked on meds and the reluctance to call these people on their addictions.

One great question for the doctor who put you on the med or vitamin: "What are you doing to get me off the meds or pill?" If the answer is "nothing" you can bet you are heading for addiction to the pill and furthermore the number of medicines you take will increase over the years.

There is a reason why 99 percent of countries have made it illegal to advertise drugs on television. It's called ethical boundaries. The ethics of selling dangerous foods has not met with ethical boundaries. Advertising and marketing seek to create addiction at its root. However, even though most advertising is unethical at best, the consumer must take the step to decide to succumb to the addiction. The circle of blaming the advertiser or pharmaceutical company becomes secondary to the ultimate decision by the consumer. We all have access to gambling, sugar, porn, alcohol, and drugs, but the path to addiction is by choice not chance.

The extension of the pharmaceutical sales approach goes to television and magazine advertisements. Even if you don't take drugs or don't believe in them, their pervasiveness in our culture has made them normal and acceptable in our culture. Imagine if cocaine or other recreational drugs became accepted as common and legal. We are going to start to see the big business of marijuana go mainstream. Many people are appalled at watching people consume recreational drugs, and we are taught how dangerous these things are to consume, until they are legalized. The framing of the substance through marketing or junk science is the key.

Look at recreational drugs. Ketamine, with a street name "Special K," is an animal tranquilizer and used as a recreational drug. The drug may also be effectively used for conscious sedation purposes as well as an antidepressant. A 2012 study from the journal *Science* found that ketamine may help stimulate the growth of synapses in the brain, and beneficial effects of the drug on people with chronic depression can occur within hours. "The rapid therapeutic response of ketamine in treatment-resistant patients is the biggest breakthrough in depression research in a half century," Ronald Duman, professor of psychiatry and neurobiology at Yale University, said in a statement.

Ecstasy has been shown physiologically to help treat people with post-traumatic stress disorder. It releases large amounts of the chemicals serotonin and oxytocin in your brain, creating feelings of relaxation and euphoria.

Magic Mushrooms (psilocybin) produce hallucinations. There's also some evidence that small amounts of psilocybin can relieve the symptoms of cluster headaches, obsessive-compulsive disorder, and depression.

Cocaine is an excellent local anesthetic and is an effective vasoconstrictor to help stop bleeding. Cocaine and the coca plant have anesthetic properties as well as a laxative and help with motion sickness and other ailments. While modern medicine has discovered much safer treatments for most of these conditions, the drug is still occasionally used as a topical anesthetic for eye, nose and throat surgeries. It has recently also been used as a topical treatment applied to the upper palate of those who suffer from severe cluster headaches.

Heroin is one of the most potent pain relievers. The National Health Service (NHS) in Britain recommends giving it to people in extreme pain, people in surgery and women in labor.

LSD used for alcoholics. A study done 50 years ago showed that recovering alcoholics are much less apt to drink excessively, and some even stopped drinking entirely for several months. Six tests were done on over 500 participants, all based on administering a single dose of acid. The LSD made the patients feel more confident, happy and satisfied with their lives, decreasing the feelings that led most of them to abuse alcohol in the first place. The effects lasted for about six months; at which point, if LSD were legal, the patients would be able to return to a treatment clinic for another dose, repeating the process until they were able to transition into (relative) sobriety.

My point in addressing this is not to encourage the use of these drugs, it is to show how subjective their use is, and how to narrow the range between legal and illegal. My point is they are close to the same except the dealer and ability to use credit cards and have your insurance pay for one.

Look at some drugs that are prescribed by doctors today. For Attention Deficit Hyperactivity Disorder (ADHD), patients have prescribed the purest form of methamphetamine: Ritalin or Desoxyn, the purest form of meth. It is also prescribed to obese people for fast, short-term weight loss. One of the most surprising uses for amphetamines is the use of the drug to help stroke victims recover more quickly. A study by the Karolinska Institute of Sweden has shown that the treatment may be very helpful for those who have been debilitated by a recent stroke.

Medical Marijuana: The drug has been shown through years of scientific research to relieve chronic pain, prevent PTSD, stimulate the appetite for people with AIDS Wasting Syndrome, control nausea, reduce intraocular pressure associated with glaucoma, treat opioid dependence, improve the symptoms of Crohn's disease and treat seizures.

In the case of street drugs, their use for medical prescription stopped because of the medical system's concern about addiction; it claims they have safer more effective drugs. The reality is that the drug companies do not have a monopoly on these natural drugs, or easily manufactured drugs, so the drug companies monopolize them and make billions. Sound corrupt? It is. Mainly because these drug companies own our lawmakers and judges.

Medical literature has shown that street heroin is much safer than the synthetic opiate oxycodone. Unfortunately, the federal government's complete ban on the drug prevents hospitals and other medical facilities from using the substance, when it is proven to be an effective and safe pain management option. The result is a crisis of oxycodone addiction. The pharmaceutical cartel makes enormous money.

Ritalin is the purest form of methamphetamine and has also created havoc by addiction yet still is prescribed and profited by the pharmaceutical cartel. The purpose of stating these facts is to help put into perspective the pharmaceutical delivery and how consumers pay the consequence through dependency and addiction. Are we blaming? Not really. It's both corruption and complacency. Without the addict buying, the dealer goes broke; it's a balance of exposing both.

The word addiction is almost like the word cancer. It has such negative connotations. The association is either one of shame and lack of self-control or pity for their disease. The goal is to give the word addiction a neutral meaning by not adding stigma. Instead, calling it for what it is: 1. A strong need to engage in an activity, substance, or thing that is harmful. 2. A strong need to participate in an activity, substance, or thing that is rewarding. The strong need is either a benefit or harm. In the case of consuming toxic stimulation substances, the net effect is harm. If the strong need to engage produces a net positive result we call this a benefit.

I have worked with many addicted people. In listening to the reasons for drinking excess alcohol, I have heard many positive reasons for consuming alcohol. "It makes me more confident." or "I laugh more." or "It relieves stress." or "I get better sales, and close more deals." I agree with these statements and ask the person what the net effect is of their choices. They start to realize that the short-term gain received is far less than the long-term costs.

Short-term gain over long-term potential is the cardinal sin in business. Looking for shortcuts while ignoring the long-term is a formula for failure. With the alcohol consumption we can see the short-term benefit of making more sales, but if the cost is a divorce, lost job, or increased medical expenses, it should become evident that the behavior should be avoided at all cost. This is obviously easier said than done.

When looking at common examples of overspending or overeating sugar and refined foods or not exercising, if you are moderately educated you fully understand that these behaviors increase your risk of illness. The same applies to spending money; just a moderate amount of education allows one to fully understand that if you spend more than you make and don't save you will not be able to retire. Or that the costs of paying credit card fees and high-interest rates cause financial illness. There was a seminar teaching the average person how to become a millionaire. It wasn't the multilevel sales pitch or the real estate sales pitch. The formula was simple: save money over a long period of time... yes, that is it. The caveat: Working hard and saving money requires virtues. The same applies to most people with weight problems—consume fewer calories than you expend, and you will lose weight or maintain a healthy weight. Find the addiction and heal.

CONSUMER DRIVEN HEALTHCARE

On the heels of calling out big pharma, I'm now calling out the consumer. Both are necessary. We have heard the statement, *"Am I my brother's keeper?"* and *"You can't pay your brother's bill."*

Ultimately what you see in our healthcare, politics, legal, etc. is a true reflection of our collective consciousness. We as a society have created the systems that we have based on demand. We can rant and point out the corruptness with precise accuracy. It is through our choices and collective consciousness that we have the ability to change. The 80 percent of people who want quick fixes without making changes, receive this in our present natural and mainstream model—this is what we have been delivered in natural and mainstream medicine. The only reason we have started to see mainstream medicine do acupuncture, integrative therapy, etc., is because the consumer has demanded it. This effort is not because medical doctors want to prescribe vitamins; it is because their paychecks require it.

I have learned that the patient who comes to me bashing their medical doctor or the mainstream medical system is a challenge to work with. They are stuck until they stop blaming. It goes back to blaming McDonald's for making you sick.

What type of healthcare stands the test of time? Surgery, acupuncture, herbal medicine, chiropractic adjustments, and faith healing all have dated back thousands of years. To look at the treatments that come and go and question how they survive without science and consistent results is a deep, challenging proposal.

In reality, it is the consumer who ultimately decides what is worthy of paying for. Both modern and natural treatments have proven to be ineffective or marginally effective yet continue to profit and thrive. Is this because insurance pays for it or because it is the only option the consumer has been told is available. The most poignant reason is that the consumer—not wanting to make changes—sees value in paying for "magic." I am always in awe of the many people who are hypnotized or flattered by their own surgical procedure. Many of these people feel special in a weird way for either having needed or undergone a surgical procedure. The specialness that people experience or magical thinking that takes place is fascinating. I think it's why people are so easily sold on surgeries which are proven to be a waste of money. Think of how many times you have listened to someone talk about their surgery with pride and excitement.

This extends to government and Wall Street. Complacency allows for the CEO making 26 million dollars a year to be the norm while paying little in tax. You and I are paying that salary with very little resistance. We also are obviously okay with them paying little taxes by way of electing politicians who enable this. The same complacency allows for politicians to be purchased by lobbyists. The same complacency provides for millions of Americans to be subject to slave labor through our prison system and minimum wage. We can sit back and blame or be victim or we can own it and take it back to balance.

CAUSE AND EFFECT

This concept is profound and complicated. Our modern science, mathematics, and physics have helped in understanding cause and effect. Cause and effect can easily be manipulated by using questionable causation: Saying that I ate at Arby's and then got in a car crash, therefore, Arby's causes car crashes. We are well aware that this is nonsense. We can say that I ate McDonald's every day last year and gained 80 lbs. We can say that the cause of the weight gain was the McDonalds I ate. The emotion or vice that led to eating at McDonald's is also a cause. In healthcare, finances, etc., we don't see cause and effect addressed much these days. You spend more than you make—you have no money—is an easy example of cause and effect. However, the cause of overspending is directly related to virtues and/ or a lack of self-control: keeping up with the Jones.

What is profound is that when we look for the cause, we are looking for explanations and answers. On the superficial level, many people ask their doctors, "What causes my PMS/cancer/thyroid problem?" The customer is satisfied with *"we don't know"* answers or believe that it's luck, chance or genetics. The customer obediently stops questioning. When we openly and persistently ask *why* we will most certainly be given answers—ask, and you shall receive. Are we asking the correct question?

A friend of mine has spent his career in the corrections area helping those caught breaking the law, using drugs, and with alcohol reform. He has observed the direct cause and effect relationship in the behavior of the majority who fail versus the small percentage of those who change their behavior and reform/heal. With confidence, this man can predict outcomes based on cause and effect behavior.

Epidemiological studies and the vast amount of casual research can now support the cause of most if not all medical issues. Twenty years ago when I started doing lectures, I recall citing a study from the National Institute of Health and the Attorney General both claiming that about 70 percent of all illness is related to nutritional factors. That amazed me back then and today I am amazed that all doctors don't speak this from their loudspeakers.

It gets more confusing when addressing health and cause and effect. Causality is objective and universal. Everything in our universe is subject to the order, motion, and cause and effect.

Cause and Effect: A person gets shot. The effect is a bullet hole in the person. The cause of the bullet hole is the bullet. The cause of the bullet entering the body is someone pulling the trigger. The cause of someone pulling the trigger: fear, drugs, etc. The cause of the fear: anger.

With your health issue(s):

Primary Cause of Poor Nutrition
- Vice - behavior governed by vice, (i.e. lazy, glutton, fear guilt)
- Addictions
- Stress

Secondary Cause of Poor Nutrition
- Intake - Poor food supply, poor food choices
- Excess - Overstimulation
- Absorption/Assimilation - inflammatory bowel disease, fatty liver, congested kidney… alcohol excess
- Increased Demand - growth spurt, activity, many chronic illnesses and recovery from weight loss
- Increased Losses - kidney disease, diabetes
- Toxins/Stimulants - alcohol, drugs, disease, environmental pollution

Effect of Poor Nutrition
- Cancer
- Heart Disease
- Alcoholism/drug addiction
- Diabetes
- Osteoporosis
- Arthritis

CHOOSING MEDICINE & ENABLING

Our medical system has mastered enabling. By telling patients, "We don't know why or how your condition came to be" or stating that their condition is genetic, chance or bad luck. This enables the same behaviors, choices and beliefs that created the condition. When any doctor tells you that they don't know what caused the condition, insist that they learn the nutritional and lifestyle conditions that are at the root of the condition they claim do not have a cause. You are paying them to know. Even modern medical studies claim that the majority of illness is attributed to diet and stress. There are thousands of studies linking lack of exercise to illness; there is research showing the connection between emotions and personality traits linking to illness. It is the choice of the doctor to read pharmacological studies instead of nutritional studies.

When a person is not respecting the principles of health or the complete paradigm and they get sick, our medical system confuses the patient by giving them positive reinforcement. The patient receives attention and sympathy, being told that the condition is not their fault.

We get confused with the strong aspects of our medical system that cloud our vision of health. There is no doubt that our modern medical system has excelled at emergency care and temporarily masking pain and other symptoms. Natural medicine does the same. With these successes, many people have become believers in the whole package, and worse, believe that emergency care somehow equates to healthcare.

There is a godlike persona that medical providers seek to attain from their patients. From the white coats to long waits in the waiting room, to nurses building up doctors as being "god." Understand that this is all a part of a conscious marketing script that our medical system has mastered. Doctors strive for patient compliance. When a doctor or any practitioner achieves this superiority over the patient, the doctor becomes all-knowing and usually receives excellent compliance. This guru, godlike persona must stop. Doctors are not above their patients. Many sick people believe that their health lies in the hands and treatments of these "godlike" practitioners. In a complete healthcare system, it requires that doctor and patient be equal. What doctors and medicine do is not mystical. Ironically, the root of this is many people's subconscious needing to be taken care of by a father figure or guru.

The medical field is a very competitive business. Mainstream medical doctors are acutely aware that their patients can quickly go to natural doctors and vice versa. Why do you think many medical doctors are not supportive of natural care? Simply put, medical doctors are either threatened or ignorant about what they do not support. The same applies to natural doctors who bash or don't support mainstream medical doctors.

It is very concerning if a medical doctor does not support natural therapies that have withstood the test of time—being more than 2000 years old and are proven not to be harmful. Just as it concerns when natural doctors do not support the medically proven modern treatments.

The underlying lesson is to differentiate that these therapies that do work are still relief, yet require a change in one's behavior to lead to healing.

HOW COMPETITIVE IS HEALTHCARE?

Stop calling yourself a patient! You are a customer. Do you realize that the medical news you watch is driven by the press releases put on by medical? Drug companies and the medical system send out press releases that appear to be news but are in fact advertisements. The same applies to most other "health alerts" or "news." Wise people realize that most TV is propaganda. The talk shows that have movie stars as guests are advertising their movies and you are paying to watch advertisements. The correlation of successful people with decreased television watching has been proven time and time again. A whopping 75 percent of the ads sold on CNN news channel is for big pharmaceutical.

Is modern medicine scientific? Is natural medicine scientific? The physiology, biochemistry, neurology, etc., found at the foundation of understanding how the body works, are very scientific. The treatments of abnormal physiology, biochemistry, and neurology ARE NOT SCIENTIFIC.

There are countless claims by modern medical practitioners that natural medicine is unscientific. Many of these claims have a foundation. In response, the natural practitioners correctly claim that modern medicine is equally unscientific and further claim that modern medicine is dangerous. It is difficult for the layperson to judge the validity of these claims.

Which form of medicine is scientific, or are neither scientific? Which form of medicine is safe? Why is there such a gap in ideology between the two forms of medicine?

Modern medicine has succeeded in minimizing the validity of natural doctors through use of the media. Below is convincing documentation that the current medical claims of natural medicine being unscientific is complete hypocrisy based on the fact that modern medicine itself lacks credible scientific proof. The purpose of outlining this is not to show that natural is a more scientific and better choice of healthcare, but rather to put both forms of medicine on a level playing field.

Both modern medicine and ancient natural medicine lack the credibility to claim the term "scientific." Many are not aware that the American Medical Association (AMA) was found guilty of a conspiracy to eliminate the chiropractic profession. Until 1983, the AMA held that it was unethical for an MD to associate with an unscientific practitioner, and labeled chiropractic an unscientific cult. The giant AMA held a quack campaign against the growing chiropractic profession. The purpose: to eliminate competition.

Even though I have claimed that there are no conspiracies to undermine healthcare, the US courts found that the American medical system did, in fact, conspire to eliminate the competitive profession of chiropractic. I stick with the conclusion that the individuals involved are corrupt. Chiropractic has not been alone in the competitive business of healthcare. The monopoly-seeking AMA also sought to destroy the credibility of homeopathy and osteopathy in an attempt to eliminate the competition.

It is documented that the AMA banned the practice of MDs consulting with homeopathic practitioners. It did the same with Doctors of Osteopathy (DO). Later, the AMA embraced Doctors of Osteopathy and has included them in the mainstream medical model. Interesting to point out that the DO became no threat once they joined forces with the MDs. One of the biggest ironies is the fact that the AMA has sought to discredit homeopathy while at the same time validating vaccines. Vaccines are based upon the same "like-cures-like" model of homeopathic. A monopoly in mainstream medicine is good only for the bottom line of the medical doctor's practice and in no way benefits the patient. The purpose of bringing these facts to your attention is to show the competitive nature of healthcare, and how the AMA has unethically used the word "science" to sell its behavior in attempting to eliminate competition. It is not at all flattering that a business would attempt to eliminate its competition illegally as opposed to beating them by being better than them. There is a place for both medical doctors and natural doctors. What is difficult is filtering out the place for medical doctors and the place natural doctors.

Can you imagine a world without business competing for market share? Think about having only one television manufacturer. Would they have been challenged to provide a larger, flatter television, with better resolution, for a better price if no other manufacturer was competing for business? Competition pushes for better answers and keeps prices competitive. Medicine is a business no different than a beverage business (like Coke and Pepsi), cell phone business or any other business. In this case, the medical system went far beyond competition into illegal activity.

Would it be fair for Coke to make up things about Pepsi to destroy the competition? Coke is free to spend more on advertising and marketing in their quest for greater market share. Coke is free to make their drink taste better to win more sales. What the medical system and pharmaceutical companies do is often unethical and illegal which is to sway customers to their field. How corrupt would it be if Coke tried to use "scientific" to build up their product and "unscientific" to degrade Pepsi's product? Or for Coke to fabricate or fund a study framing Pepsi as not healthy and Coke as healthy. Or for a cell phone company to say that "science" shows their cell phones are safe and the competitor's cell phones are unsafe. The intelligent consumer would call this out to be sure.

The modern medical system is self-governed and sets its standards for what is scientific. It is the fox ruling the hen house. The irony of the medical system calling the chiropractic profession, homeopathy, and osteopathic unscientific is the old elementary school rebuttal to name calling: "What you say is what you are, or I know you are but what am I?" Is modern medicine scientific? Most people may respond with an emphatic YES! The facts prove modern medicine is not scientific.

Mainstream medicine is NOT scientific; please don't take 200 years to change your belief on this matter. Ask questions. If you are having a difficult time with this statement do your research and prove what I am saying to be wrong. The purpose for my going on at length to explain the lack of scientific basis of modern medicine is to help you move to the next level—to help you take back your power and to encourage you to start asking questions about where health comes from and how to heal. My intent and goal are to question both medical and natural care.

A study from the Journal of Internal Medicine concluded that only 14 percent of the recommended treatments are based on sound scientific evidence. A study by the U.S. Office of Technology Assessment concluded that only 10 to 15 percent of conventional medical procedures have any basis in science.

The journal *Nature* reported that 88 percent of major studies on cancer that have been published over the years could not be reproduced to prove their accuracy. The author of the review and former head of cancer research at Amgen C., Glenn Begley, was unable to replicate the results of 47 of the 53 studies he examined—a reasonable conclusion that the cancer research and treatments are built on a house of cards.

Dr. Robert Mendelsohn, MD—who has devoted his career to opening up the channels about mainstream medical systems' flaws—states: "I no longer believe in Modern Medicine. I believe that despite all the super technology and elite bedside manner...the greatest danger to your health is the doctor who practices Modern Medicine. I believe that Modern Medicine treatments for disease are seldom effective and that they're often more dangerous than the disease they are designed to treat. I believe more than 90% of Modern Medicine could disappear from the face of the earth... doctors, hospitals, drugs and equipment —- and the effect on our health would be immediate and beneficial .... Modern Medicine can't survive without our faith, because Modern Medicine is neither an Art nor a science. It is a religion."

Another medical doctor exposes the same reality:

"Most patients probably assume that when a doctor proposes to use an established treatment to conquer a disease, he will be using a treatment which has been tested, examined and proven. But this is not the case. The savage truth is that most medical research is organized, paid for, commissioned or subsidized by the drug industry (and the food, tobacco and alcohol industries). This type of research is designed, quite simply, to find evidence showing a new product is of commercial value. The companies which commission such research are not terribly bothered about evidence; what they are looking for are conclusions which will enable them to sell their product. Drug company sponsored research is done more to get good reviews than to find out the truth."——Dr. Vernon Coleman MD

Modern medicine has used the word "efficacy" to sell the drug or treatment. Efficacy does not equate to a cure, and more importantly, it does not equate to being safe. Many drugs have efficacy in eliminating symptoms, however the dangers of putting a black piece of tape over the warning on the dashboard of your vehicle can prove disastrous.

The bottom line to scientific research is that a scientist can set up a study that shows the guise of efficacy. In other words, a drug may be effective for a very limited period of time and afterward cause various serious symptoms. For example, a very popular anti-anxiety drug called Xanax was shown to reduce panic attacks during a two-month experiment, but once the person tries to reduce or stop the medication, panic attacks can increase 300-400 percent.

To get FDA approval to market a drug, most of the studies for psychiatric conditions last only six weeks (Angell, 2004, 112). In view of the fact that most people take antidepressant or anti-anxiety medicines for many years, how can anyone consider these short-term studies scientifically valid? What is so little known and so sobering is that research-to-date has found that placebos were 80 percent as effective as the drugs—with fewer side effects (Angell, 2004, 113).

Marcia Angell, MD, author of the powerful book *The Truth about Drug Companies*, said it plainly and directly: "Trials can be rigged in a dozen ways, and it happens all the time" (Angell, 2004, 95). Conventional drugs used today are so new that there is very little long-term research on them. There are good reasons why the vast majority of modern drugs that were used just a couple of decades ago are not prescribed anymore: They don't work as well as previously assumed, and/or they cause more harm than good.

Sadly and strangely, physicians do not see that there is something fundamentally wrong with the present medical model. Instead, once an old drug is found to be ineffective or dangerous, doctors and drug companies simply assert the "scientifically proven" efficacy of a new drug. Despite this recurrent pattern, doctors are prescribing drugs at record-breaking rates.

In 2005 the volume of prescription drugs sold in the U.S. was equal to 12.3 drugs for every man, woman, and child in that year alone—compared to 1994, when 7.9 prescription drugs per year were on average purchased by every American (Kaiser Family Foundation, 2006).

If you believe that modern medicine is scientific ask your medical doctor to provide you scientific proof of the therapy or treatment in question. Watch them scramble, or use their other sales approach of guilt, shame, or superiority.

Your doctor or nurse may use a worse form of science: authority, fear, shame or guilt! Using the powers of being a doctor to ask you to follow their advice is simply the blind leading the blind.

To put the term "scientific" into perspective in comparing natural and mainstream medical, it can be said that both are unscientific and at the same time have a scientific basis. Observations and clinical trials produce a lot of scientific data. There are not many "proven" treatments in each medical field. There are some therapies and pills that produce symptom suppression very consistently. To use the term PROVEN TO CURE you must have proof. That word is often not used in both professions for good reason.

What about natural practitioners' ethics and scientific basis? Many natural practitioners push past ethical boundaries in the same ways by conducting "scientific" research that is biased to what they are selling and even going past ethical barriers and committing fraud. Often natural doctors are selling unnecessary and frivolous care similar to the modern medical care.

Question the beliefs you hold about mainstream and natural medicine. Putting all the cards on the table and showing the limitations of natural and medical practices will give you a clean slate to build your own belief system about healthcare.

Continue to respect natural and modern medicine but not worship it. Accept that neither is truly scientific, yet both are based upon an art or clinical experience. And most important, your health lies in your hands.

Again, the purpose of bringing up the battle over "scientific" is to show the hypocritical, competitive animosity in the health professions and show that neither is truly scientific. The point is to show that natural medicine and modern medicine are the same in these respects. They are involved in a fight that nobody wins and in a fight where no one is right because both professions' paradigms are not governed by a solid foundation.

In conclusion, one may find that both forms of medicine are unscientific and strive to create a religion out of their practice. With that said let's look at the bottom line—results! What is confusing is that biochemistry, physiology, anatomy, etc. are very scientific. The shortcoming is failing to address this science with cause and effect, and mind and body.

What other profession do you pay for services without the result being guaranteed or even having satisfaction with results?

Both forms of medicine achieve results in many areas of their practice. The great challenge is sifting through what does not work, what is toxic, what is dangerous, what is snake oil, and what is a waste of time, money and energy.

Many conditions are treatable by doing nothing, or watchful waiting. The majority are preventable by doctors educating their patients.

The word *profession* is derived from Latin meaning "affirmed publically." In the past, only three "professions" existed: divinity, law, and medicine. Today, the meaning of profession claims it is a paid occupation, especially one that involves prolonged training and a formal qualification.

In summary, if you accept that only 20 percent of treatments are effective and/or necessary that means that four in every five times you opt for the treatment you are not getting it. What does this mean? Simply that you are wasting time, money and energy. Or call it an expensive groundhog's day.

A question I ask myself or you may be asking is how did we get to this point? Let's go back to the center of the universe belief. Those who respected the belief of Earth as the center of the universe functioned within that limiting belief. The same applies to the present. We are functioning but not healing with these beliefs.

MEDICAL PRACTICES THAT NEVER WORKED

Prasad and his colleagues evaluated 1,344 original articles published in the *New England Journal of Medicine* between 2001 and 2010. Of the 363 articles that investigated established medical practices, 146 (40.2 percent) found the practices to be ineffective, while 138 (38 percent) reaffirmed the practices. The remaining 79 articles (21.8 percent) were inconclusive — in other words, they couldn't determine if the practices were effective or not.

The 146 medical reversals "weren't just practices that once worked and have now been improved upon," Prasad states. "Rather, they never worked. They were instituted in error, never helped patients, and have eroded trust in medicine." Examples of these reversals include the following:

- Using stents for the treatment of stable coronary artery disease
- Prescribing hormone therapy to postmenopausal women to protect against heart disease
- Routinely installing a pulmonary artery catheter for patients in shock
- Using the drug Aprotinin during heart surgery
- Prescribing COX-2 inhibitors (Celebrex, Vioxx) for inflammation and pain
- Urging people with diabetes to adhere to very strict blood sugar targets
- Treating osteoarthritis of the knee with arthroscopic surgery
- Routinely screening older men for prostate cancer with the prostate specific antigen test (PSA)

Newly established medical practices often prove to be ineffective, study finds.

By Susan Perry | 07/31/13 : A Decade of Reversal: An Analysis of 146 Contradicted Medical Practices Vinay Prasad, MD Andrae Vandross, MD Caitlin Toomey, MD Michael Cheung, MD Jason Rho, MD Steven Quinn, MD Satish Jacob Chacko, MD Durga Borkar, MD Victor Gall, MD Senthil Selvaraj, MD Nancy Ho, MD Adam Cifu, MD published online 22 July 2013.

Effective Medical, Natural and Psychological Treatments:
Short List

Medical

Setting broken bones & sutures

Stroke intervention

Cardiovascular intervention for heart attack

Surgery for spleen and appendix (sometimes)

Eye surgeries

Hip or knee replacement

Fecal transplantation

Kidney Dialysis - Diabetic therapy

Natural:

Therapeutic Fasting* (not a treatment)

Food Supplements* - Enzymes, Herbs, minerals, some oils *Most are overused or incorrectly prescribed.

Some acupuncture treatments - for pain relief

Some laser therapy

Some chiropractic treatments - symptom relief - pain relief

Some physical therapy modalities - Ultrasound, EMS, etc.

Shoulder and hip dislocation

Psychological

Cognitive Therapy

EMDR Therapy

Schema Therapy

Cross Crawl

Behavioral Therapy

Biofeedback

DOGMATISM

Dogmatism (defined): *Making principles or beliefs as undeniable truth without the open mind to consider evidence, fact, and logic that supports a different view.*

Dogmatists refuse to change changeable views. This applies to the surgeon who is dogmatically opposed to an important study proving his surgery is only for his benefit, or the natural doctor similarly providing unnecessary treatments. When confronted with new information or even different ideas, the knee-jerk person is resisting for two reasons: 1. Making us uncomfortable with past custom. 2. Humbling ourselves on being wrong. I accept this as the norm, not the exception. It is why I have included Upton Sinclair's quote multiple times in this book. It is why we address both natural and medical approaches using dogmatism.

It is through spending trillions on the wrong map that may tend to humble a small percentage of us to change.

Many doctors (most) respond to questions by customers dogmatically by creating the feeling of intimidation or acting superior to the customer asking logical or inquisitive questions. This often leads to complacency and paralysis.

We must extend this far beyond health and relationships; the dogmatism that is rooted in the "us versus them" mentality is a macrocosm of body/mind. When we see liberal versus conservative, Christian versus Islam, black versus white, east versus west, we are simply projecting. Dogmatism is the projection, and it can make us be stuck on believing that external forces cause our ill health. There is a correlation between higher dogmatism and unhappiness.

In step two of the workbook, it addresses your view of the world. The issues and projections held in these areas affect your whole health. The first step in dealing with your dogmatic position is to be open to saying "I don't know," or "I am open to changing my mind," or "I made a mistake."

The personality traits of the dogmatic are fear, anger and anxiety-based. The subconscious trait is projected outward to protect the person from these painful traits or feelings.

In health, dogmatism plagues the anti-vaccinators and the pro-vaccinators. Only the healthy can see both sides. In politics, dogmatism plagues both staunch supporters of either political view with a rigidity that does not allow dualism. Keep going to the next level with country versus country. Religion versus religion. This level of separation on a grand level is a mirror to the separation of our health and relationships.

PHILOSOPHY VS. SCIENCE VS. RELIGION

Debates on vaccines, surgery, acupuncture, and homeopathy mostly go unresolved because of the distinction between philosophical, scientific, religious and political dogmatism. If we don't lead with facts but rather with dogmatic beliefs, the result is a refusal to change.

Aristotle, the Greek Philosopher, teaches moving first to understand the science of natural bodies and physics, and then moving to the science of mind or soul. This is saying that the masculine form must be coupled and supported with the feminine. If one were to study philosophy—with the goal to create clarity with critical open thinking while examining old beliefs—we would see a very different medical system. Otherwise stated we must start with the science of physiology and microbiology to understand the cause of a viral illness then connect this with the mental aspect.

If we don't understand the purpose of illness from a biological framework how can we possibly not be dogmatic? The fundamental problem with natural and mainstream medicine is the refusal to accept science and biology incorporated with illness as purposeful—both are stuck on the germ theory.

If science is applied in both medical fields the doctor approaches the patient with clinical research, valid studies, and basic biology, physiology, microbiology, immunology, etc. If all doctors utilized these basic approaches we would see a lot less wasted dollars spent; we would also empower the patient to take charge and understand cause and effect. I am not saying that a doctor should not use methods that are "unproven." If medical and natural doctors only utilized proven techniques, we would not be able to "practice" on patients to find out what works and doesn't.

VACCINES ARE A POLITICAL
NOT A HEALTH STANCE

In understanding the germ theory and understanding homeopathy, you can make an informed decision on vaccinating. If you believe in the beautiful science behind vaccinations, you cannot insult it or not believe in homeopathy. It would be the same as believing in an airplane's ability to defy gravity while questioning a helicopter's ability to defy gravity. Both vaccines and homeopathy are founded on like-cures-like, with vaccines aiming to prevent illness and homeopathy to cure illness. Both get weak or inconsistent results because the more critical question is not being asked: how is the immune system functioning? The airplane uses lift-thrust-force and drag to create lift; the helicopter uses spinning to generate lift and the result is the same. To say that one doesn't fly is silly; same applies to saying one doesn't work and the other does for vaccines and homeopathic. Air travel is undisputed as one of the safest modes of travel. The plane will fly all the time if the conditions allow. Vaccines and homeopathy are not consistent with the results they deliver because the conditions often don't allow.

For those who believe in vaccines and even remotely understand the science behind them cannot—without openly admitting to being hypocritical and ignorant—be concerned about a non-vaccinated person in their midst.

Many informed customers of political healthcare choose not to put these vaccines in their body because of how they are processed and preserved. Or because injecting a virus directly into their bloodstream is not natural. I would personally be more open to vaccines delivered in a throat spray or topical form as mimicked in nature.

In the past, vaccines were grown on monkey proteins, and this proved to be dangerous; people are still concerned about the quality of today's protein, or the mercury used to preserve these vaccines. These chemicals have been shown to cause long-term health problems. The bottom line is that it is a choice to put this vaccination technology into your body or your infant's body. Others choose the vaccine for the connection of the weakened virus possibly helping in the prevention of disease.

If you believe that the non-vaccinated person increases your risk of illness you are duped by medical propaganda and need a class in microbiology-immunology.

If you have ever had a political discussion with a person of an opposing view, it is sometimes like talking to a wall. The vaccination issue is similar with respect to the wall. In politics, different aspects become more about attitude, belief, or tribal instinct and less about science. Those making the vaccination issue a religion ignore science and the terrible flaws of the germ theory. If you ignore herd immunity, cycles, and evolution of bugs, then it is impossible to resolve the debate on vaccinations. I have found that when discussing the vaccine issue with medical doctors, and only discussing science-based facts, the discussion shifts to an emotional one.

Again this section is not a debate. Examine the map and belief you have on the magic. Be an informed customer when paying money for things you put into your body.

The emotions and blame run high in both situations: the child being brain damaged or killed as a result of the vaccine side effect or the child being paralyzed by polio or killed by a virus. Both situations are missing the mark by blaming the proximate cause of the bug or vaccine. Yes, the judge and jury may agree that it was the vaccine that caused the harm or the virus that did. If you get stuck there, I believe resolve is difficult or impossible.

This book has hopefully weakened the foundation (house of cards) that natural and mainstream has built on the magical thinking of external care.

I recall years ago asking a "victim" mother why the vaccine damaged her child while hundreds of thousands were not? She was stuck on being a victim and blaming; I could not help her. Hopefully, I planted a seed.

THE INTEGRITY OF PROFESSIONS

The true essence of a profession only works with integrity. In the past, the oaths that governed a profession were the cornerstone of the profession's integrity. It is suggested that you review the old oaths for both medicine and law and compare them to the present. As witnessed by the medical and legal professions' oaths in the past, followed by a steady distancing from the scope of these oaths, we see a deterioration of values and ideals. Both professions see a pessimistic outlook to their respective professions.

There are consistent accounts that the legal profession is compromising their professionalism for financial gain. Furthermore, the self-governed bar associations fail to adequately punish unethical practices. The preceding are the opinions and consensus of those in the law profession—not mine. In medicine, we see the same trend. Many medical doctors fail to question procedures and practices for financial gain.

As stated, studies showing that many surgical procedures are no better than doing nothing get ignored by the doctors who financially gain. It takes a good doctor to set aside their ego when their favorite treatments or procedures are challenged by their respected peers. Chiropractors and acupuncturists selling wellness care that has no science is challenged equally.

The irony is that great doctors and lawyers are control freaks. I see this as a strength. It does, however, turn into a weakness when ego overtakes that control. In the case where the doctors who performed thousands of heart or knee surgeries are questioned about the benefits, you would hope that the doctors would put away their egos to benefit future patients. The fact is that both natural and modern doctors fail at putting their egos aside.

The alternative argument is that these doctors truly believe in their hearts that what they provide is of benefit which somehow validates what they do. If the recreational drug dealer truly believes in their heart that what they provide is a benefit to their customers does it make it okay? For the: "Hey! But dealing drugs is illegal..." argument, just substitute it with alcohol distributor.

One last thought on integrity: The doctor and street dealer both have the stance that if they did not provide the drug someone else would. The professional should be held to a higher standard because of their oath and prestigious labels attached to their names.

THE BIG EGO IS CHALLENGED

"Take egotism out, and you would castrate the benefactors." — **Ralph Waldo Emerson**

Consider the reaction of the doctors who practiced and benefited from procedures proven to be ineffective. There is a consistent backlash and resistance from doctors, possibly because their egos are hurt, possibly because they will no longer gain financially from the procedure. The irony is that there is nothing stopping these doctors—who resist the evidence that their practices are ineffective—from continuing the practice on ignorant patients. This is the reality with many of these procedures and practices, including drug therapy and surgery. Why do so many doctors put tubes in children's ear, remove tonsils, conduct arthroscopic knee surgery, provide wellness care, etc., when science proves they don't work?

I am an odds person. I don't wager in Las Vegas because the odds are not in my favor. Play long enough, and you lose. When it comes to treatments, the litmus test or gold standard is: Does this procedure work? Does this pill work 100 percent of the time?

With treatments that have higher percentages of temporary relief, there is most likely a higher degree of side effects, toxicity or complications with the therapy. Otherwise said: the stronger the result, the greater the side effects or danger. (See physics section)

Death by...

Crystals	0 in a trillion—less dangerous
Homeopathy	0 in a trillion—maybe one in a trillion
Essential Oils	0 in a trillion—maybe one in a trillion
Herbs	1 in a billion
Acupuncture	1 in a billion
Chiropractic Care	1 in 10 million
Legal Drugs	450,000 preventable deaths in US every year.
Surgery (non-cardiac)	1-4 in 100

Perspective...

"US military casualties of war" The grand total of all military deaths in the history of this country, starting with the Revolutionary War, is 1,312,612.

-Whereas 10 years of modern medical treatment cause 2,250,000 deaths.

-106,000 deaths every year from pharmaceutical drugs (Starfield)

-Between 76,000 and 137,000 deaths from pharmaceutical drugs every year in hospitalized patients (Lazerou)

-In 2010, not one single person [in the US] died as a result of taking vitamins (Bronstein, et al, (2011) Clinical Toxical, 49 (10), 910-941)."

"In 2004, the deaths of 3 people [in the US] were attributed to the intake of vitamins. Of these, 2 persons were said to have died as a result of mega-doses of vitamins D and E, and one person as a result of an overdose of iron and fluoride. Data from: 'Toxic Exposure Surveillance System 2004, Annual Report, Am. Assoc. of Poison Control Centers.'"

The United States accounts for more than a third of the global pharmaceutical market, with $340 billion in annual sales followed by the EU and Japan

Journal of Patient Safety — between 210,000 and 440,000 patients each year who go to the hospital for care suffer some type of preventable harm that contributes to their death.

Out of the **783,936** annual deaths from conventional medicine mistakes, approximately 106,000 of those are the result of prescription drug use [1]. According to the Journal of the American Medical Association, two-hundred and ninety people in the United States are killed by prescription drugs every day [4]. - See more at: http://www.collective-evolution.com/2013/05/07/death-by-prescription-drugs-is-a-growing-problem/#sthash.VTForEpR.dpuf

36,284 from traffic accidents

Everything has a risk:

Most relief treatments have side effects; when the risk is relatively low compared to the reward, we consider this effective and safe.

Exercise is one of the most effective preventive measures yet people die doing it. Keep the following stats in perspective to natural therapy (very similar), compared to modern medicine, which are drastically higher.

Dr. Thompson's studies and others show that the chances of sudden death are about one in every 15,000 to 18,000 exercisers per year. That comes to one death for every 1.5 million exercise bouts.

- One death per 17,000 men who exercise vigorously 1 to 19 minutes a week
- One death per 23,000 men who exercise vigorously 20 to 139 minutes a week
- One death per 13,000 men who exercise vigorously 140 or more minutes a week
- The same can be said about eating USDA foods. It is estimated that 7000 people each year die from foodborne illness.

We shouldn't stop eating or exercising, rather, let's be educated on making these numbers insignificant for the rest of our lives. When people get desperate they often take greater risks, like drugs or surgery. When validating a therapy for results it is not practical to justify the effects without addressing the costs. The analogy is repeated. A business has money troubles, it seeks a loan; however, the loan interest rate is ridiculously high, let's say 800 percent. The symptom of not having money goes away however the cost of the interest kills the borrower. The cost of borrowing the money is greater than the initial benefit (chemo, radiation, etc.).

Many medical protocols can be compared to an 800 percent interest rate. The cost of not looking at the true cause is much greater than the symptom relief. The same applies to the obvious toxic drugs and surgery.

When it comes down to your condition or illness, what is the success of the treatment or procedure in question? Does it have a 60 percent success rate or a 20 percent success rate? These are the numbers that have meaning, yet it is still confusing because many procedures and pills can mask or change symptoms. In masking and changing symptoms, how long does it take for a new symptom to take its place or the old one to manifest itself again?

Some medical procedures have no side effects, most of these coming from natural medicine. If the procedure has no side effects and a greater than 51 percent success, I am excited that this procedure is aiding in eliminating interference or aiding in allowing the body to heal.

If the procedure or pill has harsh side effects and greater than 80 percent success, I consider it a cure that buys someone time—at the same time explaining that we are just kicking the can down the road.

Medicine is further complexed by the fact that emotions, feelings and other motives surround the healing and illness process. The placebo and nocebo effects are a large part of mainstream and natural.

Can you turn a raisin back into a grape? The answer is no. When it comes to your health, you can't reverse some of your health conditions. With that said, modern medical and natural medical have some sound practices and treatments. Surprisingly though, many conditions are reversible... from brain injury to diabetes, heart disease, and some cancer.

If you have a gunshot wound or broken bone, there is no better place to be than in the hands of an experienced modern medical doctor. Accordingly, there are some medical emergencies that are best addressed naturally.

Pharmaceuticals, vitamins, and other supplements are effective at addressing painful or problematic symptoms. With very few exceptions the intended use of all of these pills is limited and temporary. The average intended use is between three and six months. Antidepressants are an easy example. The symptoms that antidepressants suppress will manifest by the action of the drug after six months of use. Pain medications, blood pressure medication and hormone replacement therapy all cause depletion of crucial nutrients while suppressing symptoms.

FIX ME, DOC

"Great Empires die of indigestion" — Napoleon

I am never without awe when a misdirected patient says "fix me doc" or says their doc fixed them. (I am aware that some say this jokingly, however, review The Course In Health Workbook Step 1). This type of thinking makes me think about those who want to purchase a college degree by mail or get a payday loan to solve their money problems. What a relief! You save time and money not having to go to school for four years. Bang! You have a degree. Fortunately, it doesn't work that way, and you are required to do the work and spend the time and money to get the education.

I have also heard patients claim that their chiropractor, MD, acupuncturist, etc. "saved them." The relationships formed in these cases and the genuine connections are real and in no way should be discounted. At the same time, the doctor is not a magician or miracle worker. No exceptions.

Have you ever thought that most people do not put the same expectations they have on healthcare results as they do other businesses or professions they seek? Ask yourself why? The simple answer is that if you seek guaranteed healthcare, you must be open to making changes; otherwise, the relief care cycle is acceptable.

If someone is having a stroke or heart attack the best place for them to be is in the ER getting treatment to stop the bleeding. The same applies to bone breaks and a small list of other conditions. However, it is essential to understand that the treatment is not a miracle, but simply a way to provide relief to your body for what it is unable to produce at that time. The treatment does nothing to heal the cause even though it prolongs life.

This section is difficult to navigate. I am saying that yes medical treatment can do amazing things and there is a place for these treatments, but still emphasizing that these treatments are *not* miracles. The treatment is just kicking the can down the road. The only miracle is true healing. If during these treatments the person **changes** and heals from internal means, then they chose a higher path.

I am simply asking that the patient/customer of health give the same credit to the treatment as an athlete gives to their coach. It is encouraged to have feelings of deep gratitude towards the coach, teacher or doctor for their support, but it's when you make the doctor, coach, guru, healer, drug or mechanic your God that causes separation and makes healing impossible.

BIG WORDS AND SEPARATION

Going back to the sales approach of practitioners—most professions seek the same posture. For example, the medical and legal professions created language in their fields to distance themselves from the lay people. They speak a different language to intimidate and discourage lay people from doing their own work. These types of strategies assure compliance and revenue.

Like our medical system, our legal system has lost sight of its purpose in striving for dominance and financial gain. Sadly our legal system is more about attorneys making money through billable hours then it is about solving legal issues. In time it will self-correct.

Fortunately, healthcare is self-correcting as we speak: self-correction in the form of patients (now customers or partners) starting to ask for a clear distinction between relief and healing. And more importantly, acknowledging that all "sick" systems return to homeostasis or self-correct—from the Roman Empire to a company like Enron. Self-correction occurs by either improving with time or dying with the natural competition. Self-correction is like the volcano or the forest fire. All systems self-correct over time.

On one of Pope John Paul II's visits to the United States, he required medical attention. When the attending physicians examined him and were ready to provide their diagnosis (in our medical system the language used is mostly Latin), they could not because the Pope spoke Latin, so doctors scrambled to give the Pope a diagnosis that seemed more foreign by not using Latin translations. By using a foreign language, the medical system appears more mystical and challenging to navigate on one's own; again the medical providers are separating themselves from the patient or client. Wouldn't you think that if the medical provider or attorney had their hearts in the right place they would not seek separation, but unity? The simple conclusion: We are brainwashed that we require the doctor or lawyer. The reality is that a doctor or other professional can save us time by directing us to a different path; instead, through inducing fear on the customer and or maintaining a god-like authority, they create a need for their own services.

If we call the condition "colitis" versus an inflamed gut, it is because it sounds more scary, or foreign. When something is foreign or scary or external we seek help in translation and also seek support for the fear. What if the doctor did not scare or alienate the patient? In that case, the patient could focus their attention on addressing the cause of the inflamed gut, and seek guidance and education on the cause.

SECTION 7

THE PLACEBO IS YOUR BEST FRIEND

Placebo: a substance, treatment or pill with no physiological effect given to a person that psychologically impacts the person to create physiological effect. Otherwise known as a sugar pill.

Nocebo: a substance, treatment or pill with negative effect on health that psychologically impacts the person to create physiological effect by way of explanation of negative outcome.

The placebo is real and valuable to show how powerful the internal really is. The placebo exists in natural and mainstream medicine. Studies using placebo have proven the ineffectiveness (quackery) of many medical and natural practices: from stents in the heart to arthroscopic knee surgery, to shoulder surgery, to the many outlandish claims made by multi-level marketers with their snake oil. What these studies show is two-fold: 1) How powerful the placebo is and 2) How many treatments and pills are as effective as a sugar pill.

The problem with the placebo is that the placebo is centered on taking something external. Therefore the addiction with the external pill is reinforced, or the addiction for the external treatment is being enforced. The placebo research supports many aspects of this book. It gives back the power of healing to you—the customer—if you choose it. It demystifies medicine and empowers change with one condition: that you own the internal.

Placebos show us that we don't need pills to make the chemicals our bodies make. It's the true miracle of mind-over-matter; or, the placebo shows that we think we need a pill to do what our bodies are capable of doing through placebo.

In the complex mental condition of split personalities, we see people with two or more personalities. Often this condition arises after severe mental abuse. The split personality is created to protect the individual. We have seen this portrayed in movies… one personality is Bob and the other is John. What is remarkable is that physical medical conditions are measurably different: one personality has diabetes and the other (in the same person's physical body) has no diabetic symptoms. The same has been noted for split personalities with vision differences and other conditions. This has profound implications with respect to placebos and the body connection.

The placebo effect may have a profound effect on why some of these therapies stay available. When the placebo effect has taken its hold, and results are seen, it becomes difficult to sway someone away from that treatment. If the placebo combined with the treatment in question produces results, we need to factor in the combination of the two. For example, growing a plant requires sunlight, carbon/nutrients, water, air, and the correct temperature among other things. If you give the plant everything it needs except sunlight, you would not see the miracle of growth happen. Does this mean that scientifically you can say that sufficient water, nutrients, and oxygen are not needed to produce the plant? I claim that belief and/or faith is required for all healing. Your belief may be in God or a god, a pill, a doctor, a prayer, a treatment, or a diet. When it is built on internal truths (like God or prayer), the healing lasts; when it is something external… it is temporary.

I believe that many conditions simply require the belief in your own ability to heal or your Creator's wisdom to allow for healing to occur in your physical body and spiritual mind. The problem again is that we have been told so many times that we require the treatment or the pill. What makes this further confusing is that in some instances— probably NOT yours—the pill or treatment, in combination with belief, is what is necessary to heal. The big question still remaining is what was the purpose of the condition? If all disease is a goal-oriented, biological process and the process restores us back to health, it would be short-sighted to think that healing takes place with the treatment or pill. The purpose of the illness is to get us back on track because of emotional blocks or other issues; the pill or treatment *not* addressing the emotional issue would not heal the condition.

If this opens up the idea that the placebo/belief is a cornerstone of healing we need to embrace it. Consumer-driven health has evolved by patient/customer demand. Essentially in all corners of commerce, what the consumer wants the consumer gets. We have seen this with modern medicine conforming to consumers' demands by shifting to a more natural approach to healthcare. I guarantee if the consumer did not demand that their medical doctors provide them with more natural medical ways the medical doctors would not have made their shift.

Alternative (Natural) therapy is in fact not so alternative when the data shows that approximately 50 percent of the US population uses "alternative" therapy on a regular basis. Clearly, the consumer does not see the natural practitioner as an alternative. This begs the question, is there an alternative to "natural?"

Consumer-driven healthcare at present is about avoiding pain—a purely masculine driven approach. When pain is embraced, as in natural childbirth or headaches without intervention or meds, there is no need for placebo. The ability to overcome pain is internal.

The only major setback the placebo has is that it is mostly (or possibly entirely) external and temporary and because the pill or treatment is external it makes healing and relief far apart.

The late Dr. Sarno is a medical doctor who clinically proved that most of the chronic pain people experience is a result of emotions. His entire practice involved helping those to focus on the emotions. A condition of his care was that you not be involved in any external form of care: massage, chiropractic, physical therapy, etc. The reason is that people focus on the physical symptoms instead of their emotional state. It is similar to exercise and diet If we focus on the illness and use an exercise program to fix the illness, the exercise is short lived or the fix is temporary relief. Diets become perpetual, and we fail as well.

At this point in time, the belief system of mainstream medicine is beginning to waver, resulting in negative energy transferred to the patient which we call the nocebo. The natural system has a much stronger belief system in their "go-to" external treatments. This then transfers to the patient by way of positive energy. Your thoughts are more powerful than any drug on the market. They are limited only by your own disbelief in your body/mind's ability to heal. I once heard a doctor remark, "There are no incurable conditions, only incurable people." (Dr. Robertson)

To truly grasp this statement it would connect you to the truth of your "condition" and it would redirect your attempts to overcome it. This doctor is of the new breed whose purpose is to walk with you on your journey to healing. This type of person will be brought into your life when you are ready. They will not charge money for their support. They will learn from you, as you will learn from them. They will listen to you, but not in the sense that you are perhaps expecting. Because you are equals, they will be able to refrain from judgment despite the fact that they may possess a better intellectualization of the process. Blending two minds in the search for truth has historically created a powerful "third" mind, which will shorten the journey for both. One thing I have been confronted with continually in my practice is the determination of the patient to avoid accessing their own ability to change and heal. What they are seeking from me is validation that their problem relates to their external circumstances (luck, chance or genetics) rather than accessing their own internal compass and personal belief system that is necessary for their successful healing. To be successful the patient needs to shift their thinking from the external direction of the doctor to the internal reflection that is necessary to create successful healing.

*"You were lost in the darkness of the world until you asked for light. And Then God sent His son to give it to you" (*ACIM).

I would like to interject a little story here that I hope makes you laugh, and makes you think. A passer-by was in the city late one night when he happened upon a gentleman scouring the ground underneath a street lamp, obviously in the attempt to retrieve a lost article. Wanting to help, the passer-by offered to search. In order to achieve maximum efficiency, of course, he requested information of the frantic gentleman. The gentleman was grateful for his help, and told him he was searching for his keys. The two hunted and hunted to no avail. Determined to find his keys, the passer-by questioned the gentleman as to where exactly he was standing when he lost the key ring. To his surprise, the gentleman pointed far down the street, and said without hesitation, "Over there." The passer-by was astonished. He asked why on earth, then, was the gentleman searching at this end of the block? The gentleman, without looking up, replied simply, "Because the light is so much better here." This story is a parable for the powerful drive we humans have to remain in the same state of consciousness that brought us to our problems. We must be willing to light up the dimmer areas of our understanding in order to find what we seek where we "lost" it.

Healing does not come from someone's magic touch, nor does it come from a pill. Anytime we look outside ourselves we are seeking relief versus healing. Healing is living with the focus of unity, while magic is separation which seeks external treatments.

Relief care is not healing. Relief care is either naturally or medically suppressing a symptom or providing a treatment that allows your body to heal on its own.

Both mainstream and natural offer low percentage relief care for most conditions. Antibiotics for a bladder infection or pneumonia provide relief to the immune system that was weak and allowed the bacteria to grow. The confusion must be clarified to enable you to become empowered over the germ theory brainwashing. Antibiotics can't heal a bladder infection or pneumonia because antibiotics don't address the cause of the bacterial overgrowth. No sound microbiologist or immunologist would claim otherwise. If the antibiotics kill the bugs, the immune system must step up and create homeostasis; it is why we see so many people die in hospitals hooked up to IV antibiotics while the bacteria flourish.

SECTION 8
LAWS OF THE LAND

Just because our laws allow for certain behaviors and have made some drugs legal to purchase does it mean that these drugs are okay to consume? Just because the FDA approves a drug or allows a particular food into the supermarket does it mean it is healthy? The main difference between pharmacy heroin (opioids) and street heroin is that you can purchase one with a credit card and the other you cannot. The other main difference is the one on the street is sometimes purer.

Marijuana is legal in some states; does that make it okay or healthy? The same questions apply to refined sugar, genetically modified foods, artificial sugar, pharmaceutical drugs or other street drugs like cocaine.

Travel across the globe and we see recreational drugs range from illegal to legal. Punishments for illegal use range from a slap on the wrist to the death penalty. Is it safe to say that a large reason for making these drugs legal is economical? As far as foods in our supermarkets, some countries have banned certain foods to be consumed while others allow for the consumption. Genetically Modified Foods (GMOs), Hydrogenated Oils, Brominated Oils and Bovine Growth Hormones are several examples of foods being banned in some countries. Looking into the reasons of these bans, the underlying reason is that these foods have been proven to have negative health consequences.

The question then arises why these same countries do not ban tobacco use, excess alcohol consumption, refined sugar, etc., as these items have been proven to have negative health consequences.

Facts show that pharmaceuticals and foods are regularly getting recalled or pulled from the shelves. Some are later banned. Hydrogenated oils were mainstream when many people ate margarine instead of butter. Hydrogenated oil was considered safe for 40 years and now science is warning against its consumption altogether. The same thing can be said about many legal drugs. If you would like more information you can search the internet for "black box" or prescription toxicity.

Does allowing people to have access to any food, gambling, or drug, speed up the process of healing? Why not have the government tax and profit off these destructive behaviors to help offset the heavy cost associated with them? The counterargument would be that our government and leaders need to safeguard us against these negative/ toxic things. Is the answer in the balance of allowing people to have access to drugs, tobacco, gambling, alcohol, toxic foods, etc. with full disclosure (education being the key)? If you educate people on why the sin-tax is in place on toxic things, taxing the toxic agent results in paying for what helps lead us back to health. It may not be the answer if you consider that you are your brother's keeper. If we allow people to drug themselves, gamble, etc., we as a society pay the price on a spiritual and financial level.

Often people complain about our medical system; they want to blame doctors, hospitals, and insurance companies. The reality is that our medical system has given people what it has asked for: relief care without any requirement to change one's lifestyle. I.e. Pain management at any cost.

Drug companies give you the toxic side effect warnings on the label and the television or magazine advertisement. Even though these warnings are minimized or downplayed, they still do exist.

Cambridge psychologist J.T. MacCurdy published his findings from the London England Bombings in World War II. He studied peoples' fears based upon near misses versus distant misses of bombs. He found that people experiencing near-misses are deeply affected versus those experiencing a remote miss or miss from a distance. The latter felt excited and even invincible. The optimistic side is people's ability to see the positive and be able to function. The apathy or denial should be concerning of human behavior.

If we equate this to the "remote miss" of pharmaceutical side effects—affecting someone else and not you—the result is excitement and invincibility. For the few who get the toxic medical scare or near-death experience from their prescribed drug, they are deeply affected. This psychological phenomenon is regarded as a detachment, or lack of apathy, or compartmentalization: identical to that of taking drugs; doing nothing for mass school shootings that are remote to you; identical to the apathy we experience when we hear about prisoner abuse from a distance; identical to the apathy we experience when we hear about corruption in the courts, police departments or Wall Street. Sounds deep and heavy, yet explains our apathy to change. Or the apathy and invincibility while taking drugs.

The justice/legal mindset is that of the medical mindset, we just have not connected them. Think about the legal elites that misuse the law to selectively use and exploit the law to get people off: Getting a murderer or rapist off on technicalities regarding the collection of evidence or other ways the law was not intended to be used is commonplace. Exhausting others' resources to win a lawsuit is commonplace. It is obvious that the legal system is rigged and a complete failure because it is tailored towards the rich. This book may not change that fact, yet it may change how you look at health as it relates.

The parallel is the big pharmaceutical getting away with pushing a dangerous drug through by using loopholes or shady scientific protocols. Or no accountability to the medical profession for killing millions with dangerous and unproven medication and medical treatment that are also unproven and dangerous. The outcomes are identical. Think why street drug dealers are often put away for life in prison while the drug companies and doctors giving the same drugs are protected?

The next connection we make is the billionaire getting away with paying no taxes with the same loopholes. By the way, the loopholes, laws, and lobbyist are controlled by the elite. Something the OJ's, lobbyist and benefactors should be wary of is the cost of this vice. The point being, justifying eating a toxic food, prescribing toxic drugs, taking toxic drugs because the law allows, may make you as ill as OJ Simpson.

The responsibility of the "professional" should go beyond hiding behind warning labels. Doctors who are paid generously and held in high regard should be held to a higher ethical and moral standard.

The medical doctor who aided Michael Jackson in his death is the extreme example, but I believe MOST medical doctors are equally culpable in their actions. Dr. Conrad Murray was found guilty of involuntary manslaughter (murder) for providing prescriptions drugs that caused Jackson's death. Drugs Jackson demanded.

How many doctors are not held accountable for involuntary manslaughter for the deaths caused? Close to 500,000 deaths occur yearly in the USA are due to MD prescribed drugs. These (medically caused) leading causes of death have been removed from the "lists" of top causes of death for the USA.

Unlike pharmaceutical companies, pesticide companies are not required to post warnings on produce or meat products indicating the side effects of the chemicals to your body. The same applies to food. Many have asked for cheap food, so that is what we have been given (food that is less money and cheap). Foods grown without pesticides and chemicals cost more to make in the short-term.

CHASING THE DREAM THE LOTTERY TICKET

The lottery ticket analogy to making change applies to money, relationships, and health. I propose that 80 percent of the population is sick when it comes to their health, finances, and relationships. It is fascinating to know that if you gave these 80 percent a winning lottery ticket they would squander it because of the laws of nature.

The lottery ticket thinking goes like this: If I just had more money I would be happy. Conversely, the people who do not have lottery ticket thinking believe that to be happy they need to start with being happy. When we begin with the end in mind, we see lasting success.

The lottery ticket thinking extends to the same thinking with health, work, and relationships. If I work hard enough or long enough, I will have what I need or want and will be happy. In health, it goes like this: If I do the treatment I will have no pain and be happy.

This lottery ticket scenario causes people to work more at the doing when they are not satisfied with their having. This pattern will get challenged at some point. When it does, people will look at themselves instead of money, fame or power to make themselves happy. Many people believe that the winning lottery ticket is the key to their happiness, thinking that they would be less stressed and happy if they had their house paid off or a set amount of money.

These lottery ticket winners are given the opportunity to have all their troubles vanish overnight. In reality, the unbalanced state of these "winners" is still there in the morning, the next week and the next year. A good majority of these individuals ultimately resort to drugs, alcohol or other destructive behaviors. Many lose their money. Why? Because they fail to take responsibility for their state of dis-ease and continue to blame. The winning lottery ticket could be a good thing, if you take it, look yourself in the mirror and realize that winning the lottery does not solve ANY of your internal issues.

Most people do not have the opportunity to win the lottery, and they continue to believe that the root of their stress or negative emotional state is due to their lack of money.

They do more with the belief that *doing* will allow more *having* so they can be happy or healthy. This approach to health or happiness usually happens over a long period of time. People have a list of things that they believe will make them happy, unstressed, confident, etc. These may include a home that is paid for, so much money in the bank, a certain job title, a certain house, a certain number of kids, certain clothes, furnishings or cars. They work hard to do the work to have the title or money, but when happiness or peace eludes them they look somewhere else to do more.

The lottery ticket is a great way to look at things because it is a condensed time frame in the realm of the Doing-Having-Being model. People who purchase lottery tickets believe somehow that there is something material missing in their life that would be fulfilled if they had this amount of money. Again please look back to the paradigm of external-external versus internal-internal.

As a side note, it is interesting to point out that the majority of people who purchase lottery tickets on a regular basis are less educated than those who do not. Educated people know instinctively that there are no shortcuts. Buying lottery tickets is a useless tax on the poor which the educated/healthy don't succumb to.

IS THERE A TIME TO RESIST?

Refer back to the balance and dualistic section outlining the medical system as 99 percent masculine. The Christian Science religion's stance insists on no medical intervention (few exceptions, i.e. bone break); essentially the religion upholds "never" a time to resist or fight using mainstream medicine (medicine saying "always" to medication, vaccines, chemo, etc. for everything and never tolerating pain). This religion says *never* to these treatments because the condition has come about by incorrect thinking—taking many of the same stances this book takes. I applaud and respect the internal aspect. The problem I see with the Christian Science religion is the lack of respect for the masculine form of medicine which has value. At the same time, we must acknowledge the difference between relief care versus healing.

The story that comes to mind is the guy who was so impressed with a friend who didn't have a watch, never had to set his phone for appointments, was never late for appointments, and always woke at the time he intended. So, the guy tossed his watch and did not set his alarm on his phone. What happened was chaos. He was late, causing inconvenience to himself and others. The intention of this guy to be more intuitive, spiritual or more in touch was not prudent because he was trying to be something or someone he was not. He was not accepting where he was at. Our religion teaches us to turn the other cheek and forgive. In so, there is healing and virtue. When you are at that point to be able to forgive from your heart it is of value that cannot be put into words. If you "think you" forgive someone from stealing from you *but* you are not genuinely okay with it, you are not being realistic about how you truly feel and therefore you will most likely stew or resent being wronged. This is because where you truly were at was *needing* to collect the bill.

In theory, the Christian Science religion should ban watches and clocks because the genuinely connected person should not need one. Being late is an error of thinking and should be healed with prayer.

Many years ago just out of college, I had a vehicle that I didn't carry collision insurance on. I told my stepdaughter three times not to drive the car, as I explained that the icy road conditions and her inexperienced driving were the reasons. She took the car out while I was gone, drove on an icy road she had never driven on and flipped the car. The car was totaled. I felt anger and wanted her to pay for the damage as I had no insurance. Many people told me I should just be happy that no one got hurt and I needed to let it go. Such guidance is easy to give when the advisor does not suffer any consequence.

The same applies to healthcare. If some religion, doctor or friend tells you not to get a medical treatment done because it is the right or wrong thing to do, step back; make sure you are realistic about where you are. It goes both ways: for the MD pressing you to take chemo versus the natural doc telling you not to; the MD pressing you to take a vaccine and the natural doc telling you not to. This book is in no way telling you what to do. It is giving you informed facts and a correct map to use. This book does suggest, claim and state that the existing map many use is incorrect. There is no force, shame or guilt with the choices you make for relationships, health or finances; as stated several times: either they bring you closer to your Grand Purpose or further away; either they allow for healing or make healing not possible; either they save time or not.

The Christian Scientists are correct in saying the condition starts in the mind. However, they are disrespecting the masculine form of energy; in fact, they forbid it. Healing takes place when the masculine and feminine connect. This is confusing in light of the fact that those engaged in an external treatment for a condition believe that the cause is external. That level of thinking reflects the dismal results seen with many conditions. As outlined within and supported by mainstream research, the majority of health problems are caused by nutrition, lack of exercise and stress. Realistically people are not ready to take personal responsibility and therefore need access to relief care. This is not to concede to external means; it merely proves the analogy that payday loans need to be illegal because they make healthy finances impossible. It is accepting that a loan may be helpful at certain times for certain things; however, borrowing money to get by is dangerous.

The moralist who says to forgive someone who steals from you is correct. It is a path to healing. They are also disrespecting the masculine form if they judge someone for collecting the debt. The only correct answer is the one that leads to healing and saves time. In the workbook, we address this in more detail. If someone steals from you and you choose civil remedy over forgiveness, you recover your money but the pattern continues. You find yourself in the same situation, and the stress is killing you. You may start looking at other ways to remedy the pattern and forgiveness may be the answer.

Back to the question on using medical treatment—yes, if it saves you time, or if you require to accept "where you are" (or demonstrating where you are). Is there a time to declare war, or fight when it comes to health, relationships, or finances? There is ample proof that supports a need for combative tools such as using drugs, filing a lawsuit, or fighting back. The question remains: Can Whole Health and Peace be a result of fighting? Not directly, yet I believe the indirect result may bring about healing. I propose the fight which is separation can and does result in healing if a change occurs or if enlightenment ensues while combating. It is called the gold in the womb.

The two "fighting" professions that come to mind are doctors and lawyers. Both take the stand of fighting and winning against external forces by using blame. Both professionals charge and deserve bags full of money because their jobs are mostly toxic. Many doctors and lawyers can't handle the blame and toxicity because it becomes a part of them. It is why I believe they deserve a lot of money as compensation. In no way is this stance to offer disrespect to these professions, if anything it is support and empathy. If you talk to honest veterans in these fields they would support this. Doctors and lawyers are dealing with sick people (for the most part) who are blaming.

So when is fighting in health warranted? Take for instance you or your child develops spinal meningitis and heavy dose antibiotics may help fight the overgrowth of bacteria while the immune system removes dead cells. Yes many have overcome the bacteria overgrowth naturally or others may overcome the bacterial overgrowth through faith or prayer. Yet your belief at the time is shaky. Fighting with antibiotics makes sense while you recover and take a deeper look at what caused the weakened immune state. Another example is you are diagnosed with breast or testicular cancer; you fully understand and believe that the cancer was rooted in emotions yet have beliefs that if you don't have it surgically removed you will die. Having the surgery while you internalize may be the best answer.

Is fighting warranted for simple conditions like back pain or a headache? Again this is 100 percent up to the informed customer. This book is not intended to judge any person needing external relief; it simply offers a balance with a feminine form to achieve healing. Without judgment, we should ask ourselves why we choose to cover up purposeful pain for our conditions.

There are many other examples of laws or rights being violated where fighting would help bring resolve with one underlying condition. That is to internally resolve your role in the dysfunction that created the need to fight. This is when the focus of your role is addressed throughout. Rosa Parks and Gandhi are familiar examples. The targeting of minorities requires civil rights changes through this masculine form. The corruption in government and Wall Street require the same.

The same applies to health. The key is not using these vices of fighting as a fallback. Medicine and law do not have to be toxic. It is when they are abused that they become toxic. The OJ Simpson lawyer team had knowingly used and abused the masculine form of the legal system as do many lawyers; they each justify their actions just as the drug dealers do. Sounds very harsh but it is not. Our legal system is intended to do good, just as is our medical system. Any person involved in the legal system will admit the rich get away with murder (sorry OJ). Money has corrupted the legal system and medical system. When the poor black man does not have the same means to the civil process because he is offered a public defender paid $400 to defend his crime versus the $4,000,000.00 paid by OJ... connect the dots.

"Power tends to corrupt, and absolute power corrupts absolutely. Great men are almost always bad men." — Lord Acton

Any person involved in the medical field will admit that big pharma gets away with murder—literally and figuratively. Money has corrupted the medical system. In summary, the toxicity comes from the subconscious blame that these professions use to justify their actions. A healthy form of medicine or law does exist. I have an attorney friend that is also an impeccable organic farmer. His practice of law is where the masculine form is respected, and feminine energy is allowed. There are no dilemmas and no toxicity. He uses the masculine (laws and codes) to create healthy resolution by respecting fairness and justice (feminine). In medicine, there are doctors who respect the masculine aspects of medicine and allow the feminine. These doctors are happy and congruent and they give credit to what truly allows for healing.

Growing up Catholic we went to confession on a regular basis. We would openly repent our sins and ask for forgiveness. Is sin going against our Grand Purpose? I suggest it is. Is covering up pain—or kicking the can down the road—sin? The purpose of the confessional is not to enable sin, it is the opposite. If we go against our physical well-being by drinking too much alcohol or eating junk food is that a sin? Is someone covering up those symptoms that result from these vices helping or hurting? The purpose of vices, negative emotions, and illness is to bring us back to balance or homeostasis through virtue, happiness, and wellness. I say we can't have one without the other. I also say neither is bad and both are necessary! The vice or sin is not necessary if we stay internal with our Grand Purpose. The confessional is an amazing outlet not to be used as a vice.

In the great majority of cases, the physics of peace makes the most sense. So it would seem that ancient therapies are the most logical choice we can make when choosing health.

When the spirit is to "fight" a disease with external means we are doomed to failure. If the focus is for a Grand Purpose, the results differ. It often does not matter if the approach is medical or natural. I have studied many who have had "spontaneous remission" from a cancer diagnosis. What I believe has allowed for the healing or cure of these cancer growths was the spirit in which the diagnosis was handled. Those who cure or heal share one common trait: working with, learning from or embracing their condition (whether it is cancer, heart disease, headaches or a skin condition). The not blaming, not being embarrassed, and not being ashamed of their condition has made all the difference; they have a purpose in life. This is the cornerstone of the complete paradigm. People heal with or without medical treatment.

At this point, it is again important to make the distinction between relief care (disease care) and healthcare. When I ask patients if they would like disease care or healthcare, the majority pick health. This is where the dilemma is created.

If your doctor is honest with you he will explain that disease care does not pay whatsoever. It actually costs you. The analogy goes like this: Your automobile brake indicator lights up on your dashboard. You bring it to your auto mechanic. He/she explains that your brakes are faulty or "diseased." The mechanic asks you if you would like relief care (disease care) or healthy auto care. Healthy auto care requires you to change the brake pads and rotors. The disease care takes into consideration that you don't have the time or money to do healthy auto care and consists of the mechanic putting a black piece of tape over the brake light indicator on your dashboard.

The problem is people's reluctance to change. This is a big reason mainstream medicine has gotten so technical. Forty years ago an MD would tell you to go home and rest and drink water for your cold or make yourself some chicken soup. The patient would think why did I just pay X amount of dollars for someone to tell me something so simple?

We as a culture have invested a lot of energy to not change. These areas where we refuse to change will always create conflict. Our medical system has pioneered and exploited this. If the confessional becomes a means to justify a vice, it too becomes a vice. If the drug becomes a means to justify a vice, it is a vice.

Our medical system has listened to people's desire to make the pain go away and not address the underlying issue. Our medical system has been created by the people. Our legal system is founded on resolving disputes civilly; the premise of this civility is sound and often works. When you have been wronged and seek to resolve it, the civil process provides closure.

This leads to the next question: Should the doctor treat you or not? The "center of the universe" belief system is in play.

Note on Christian Science: The mention of the Christian Science religion is not intended to offer any disrespect. The Christian Science beliefs and their courage to make a stand on true healing are virtuous. The attack they receive is almost entirely from ignorance and fear. It has been outlined in the **Denialism section** and the Center of the Universe sections.

"First they ignore you, then they laugh at you, then they fight you, then you win." —Mahatma Gandhi

Einstein stated, "Great spirits have always encountered violent opposition from mediocre minds."

I offer my clinical and personal opinion that the great spirit of Christian Science and the courage to endure the attack makes their focus real. I offer the same opinion to those who take the teachings of Jesus (Sermon on the Mount) and apply them without compartmentalization.

"If you want to make enemies, try and change something." — Woodrow Wilson

One last thought on treating alcoholics with "AA". This approach gets bleak results. Estimates are less than 10 percent with lasting results, while 70 percent of alcoholics who receive NO help succeed in their addiction. Those numbers are mind-blowing.

"There's no such thing as an evidence-based rehab. That's because no matter what you do, the whole concept of rehab is flawed and unsupported by evidence," says Dr. Mark Willenbring, former director of treatment and recovery research at the National Institute on Alcohol Abuse and Alcoholism.

The flaw with AA and most rehab is it is based upon external-external. The numbers will not change until we change to internal-internal.

The question: Does treatment stagnate or interfere with healing? I claim with every clinical bone in my body and every aspect of my gut that many, if not all, treatments create a flawed attachment to the external. This makes healing difficult. And at the same time if you require that you use external, do so without blame, guilt or fault and you will likely be compelled towards the internal with that focus.

INSURANCE DILEMMA

I am a believer in universal healthcare as a right and as a privilege, and as a component of social security and social justice; the dilemma is responsibility and entitlement with free healthcare. The majority of healthy people who have access to universal healthcare do not use or abuse it.

For some people, the worst thing for our healthcare is "health" insurance. First of all, it should be called *illness insurance*. The biggest problem with insurance is that there becomes an entitlement and/or expectation with using the policy paid for. The only thing I believe that is worse than insurance policies are insurance policies that people do not need to pay for. The two best predictors of life expectancy are average GDP (Gross Domestic Product) and education level.

If a person wants a procedure that has proven to be ineffective like arthroscopic knee or shoulder surgery—which costs money and has few side effects—is the doctor required to consider the healthcare costs that other people pay for this procedure? Perhaps the next ethical question is: Do we continue to spend more and more on healthcare expenses on a per capita basis that exceeds a nation's ability to pay or than an individual person is able to contribute in a lifetime? There is no insurance dilemma with the Internal Grand Purpose.

"There can be change without progress but not progress without change."—Anonymous

LIKE LEARNING TO PLAY THE PIANO

Like everything else in life that is worth pursuing, there are no shortcuts when working towards better health. The most expensive medical technology cannot restore a body to the person who does not respect the very basic fundamental laws of health, nor can the highest quality food supplement. Have you ever met a doctor who can take two halves of a sliced apple and make it whole again? And yet this is what we are asking our doctors to do. There is absolutely nothing any well-intentioned physician can do to overcome what we won't do for ourselves. Asking our doctors to make us healthy is just as ridiculous as asking them to learn to play the piano for us.

Whether it is learning to play the piano or learning golf, there is a valid argument that having the proper tools and coaching is essential. As detailed throughout this book, the proper tools equate to proper nutrients and also some coaching on how to prepare these foods (or possible treatments in certain circumstances). The majority of learning has to do with the person's commitment to doing the work. I started playing golf when I was 40 years old. I became hooked on the game and wanted to get better. In the process of dropping over 25 shots off my score, I came to the conclusion that the equipment and coaching had a small and notable contribution to my growth. Where the majority of my growth and mastery of the game came from was from personal factors (internal). The interesting parallel to overcoming a condition and overcoming a slice in golf is that there are so many snake oil salespeople selling the magic, "easy" cure. In healthcare, it is commonly the drug or pill. In golf, it is the purchase of a video or swing training device. The more the salesman claims it is fast, and/or easy, the red light comes on. Any golf-swing coach will tell you that the most important factor in golf above proper mechanics is repetition and work. All professional athletes have a natural talent yet there are exponentially more athletes with equal or greater talent who do not succeed.

You will see common attributes of successful athletes, musicians, business people, having: 1) self-control 2) high levels of self-efficacy.

Self-Efficacy is about Adapting, Effort, Perseverance, and Persistence.

Self-Control is the ability to control Feelings, Thoughts, Words, Actions, Habits, and Character, especially in difficult times (See The Course In Health Workbook).

The same applies to health. Those who heal or stay healthy take on the attributes of professionals in other areas. Does it mean that you need to be a pro? Absolutely not. Yet striving for perfection and high standards is a definite plus. Change the words to Grand and Purpose.

THE STEPS EXPLAINED -RADICAL CHANGES

"L.I.V.E. to Heal" = Looking Internally Versus Externally

The steps attached within guide you to The Emotion-Link and A Course in Health. More details on the first four steps are provided in this section:

STEP 1 - WORDS

"It is written, 'Man shall not live by bread alone, but by every word that comes from the mouth of God.'"(Matthew 4:4)

- Your words create your questions
- Your questions turn into thoughts (conscious and subconscious)
- Your thoughts translate to actions
- Your actions create habits
- Your habits shape your character
- Your character becomes your virtue or vice

Our words we speak out loud or internally are the start of either health or illness. Our subconscious does not know the difference between real and imagined; it's why we get a physiological response from a nightmare.

We often use words that interfere or make healing impossible. When you say I want to be healthy "but" don't have the time to… all that your subconscious, your soul, your entire being hears is the "but" that negates "I want to be healthy." Also, most challenging is the honesty required in your language to describe your health challenges.

If you say "I don't know" versus "I want to know" you have not asked therefore you have nothing to receive. "I want to know" is the start of receiving whole health or answers to anything. You will only receive answers to the questions you ask.

When you carry a lot of baggage from internal conflict and you self-sabotage health, wealth, and relationships, your language is the best guide. If you are not able to say that you are worthy of health, or if you can't say it's possible to have healthy finances, that becomes your reality. Even deeper are the inconsistencies and blame we use through words.

These self-sabotaging words we choose allow for ill health to manifest—consistent with the cause of all disease outlined. It's subconscious and powerful. By changing our words we are taking back the power.

Once you start changing your words, step 2 will become clear and you can address the words we use with judgments, thoughts, feelings, and projections.

Tell your close friends and partner your goal of eliminating these words and thank them when they point them out.

"What goes into someone's mouth does not defile them, but what comes out of their mouth, that is what defiles them." (Matthew 15:11)

Words guide our subconscious and our thoughts in obvious ways. If we say negative things when positive events happen, or don't understand the difference between permanent versus pervasive, or temporary versus specific, or if we don't understand what limiting beliefs are and how the words we use enhance the limiting belief or challenge it—we will be stuck. No matter how hard we try.

The words we use often enhance the external-external approach by empowering luck, chance or genetics, versus taking back our power by using internalized words.

Understand the difference between facts and opinions. Otherwise said: the difference between objective versus subjective. Healthy people use factual descriptions (objective).

Think of Objective/Factual words being "internal" and the Subjective/Opinions being "external". Truth/Reality versus Opinion and Judgment. The difference between observations and judgments is the key to journaling. An observation is a fact. A judgment is an opinion; our lives are full of judgments and don't allow for growth, honesty or change.

Self-judgments and projections are key: This is the shift from external to internal. All of step 1 is hinged upon honestly using descriptive words to express your judgments and conditions. Beliefs and thoughts change when we shift from external to internal.

Understanding the purpose of this and the context is key. "I enjoy the beauty of nature while hiking" versus "today was so beautiful," or "John is good because he has not done meth for 30 days," versus "I feel so good when I don't inject meth into my blood."

Changing the Rules...

Many have learned expressive dialogue (in marriage counseling or elsewhere) where you express your feelings in terms of someone else's external actions. We are going to stop that right now. This type of counsel makes victims and does not bring resolve. The only benefit is that it makes you aware of feelings you have.

You may hear the marriage counselor telling the couple to "use your words" or a mother saying the same to their child. We will use our words and use them wisely.

When I say: "I feel controlled when my wife orders my meal at the restaurant," the focus then becomes an external one and the feeling is lost in the behavior of the "controlling wife." The wife needs to change her behavior so the husband doesn't feel controlled. What I propose is a resolution for your "feelings" that shifts from external to internal. It requires the person expressing their feelings to own them by making the feelings a descriptive (internal) feeling. So if I say I feel controlled by my wife, I must commit to following up by saying "I am being controlling to feel this feeling." This concept is confusing for most people because our blaming ways have been validated for so long.

Side note: Would you rather be right or happy? You may get people to side with you on the blame game.

So how this works requires somewhat of an open mind. When a customer comes to me and says "I need help, I am depressed," I ask why they say they are depressed? They say my doctor says so. I in turn, ask if they are "depressed" 24 hours a day and 365 days of the year? They always respond NO I am just depressed when... (I am alone, or at night, etc.). I reply you are not "depressed" you feel depression at night... This shifts the word depressed to depression with a lot of positive ramifications leading to resolve. "Depressed" is external, permanent and pervasive; it is "disease" that is pretty depressing (no pun intended). The words "feeling depression" is temporary and specific—way more empowering. However, we don't stop here.

I then ask "how does a person feel depressing?" For example, if you are picked to play the part in a movie or play, I explain that to act depressing you have to change your voice/tone, posture, and entire demeanor. The conclusion is agreed that to feel depression you must "be depressing." This is the internal step. I ask the person to commit to saying "I am being depressing" every hour on the hour for the next three days by setting an alarm. After saying this a few times, most, if not all people will transform their belief on being depressed and internalize a purposeful state. Some may think this is ridiculous or simplistic. When you do this with intent along with the next three steps it is incredibly powerful.

WHY THINGS ARE NOT GOOD OR BAD...
ON THIS MAP

As stated throughout the book the physics of change requires a shift from external, harsh blame to internalizing and taking charge through gently accepting vices and pain as purposeful.

If we make the vice "bad" and the virtue "good" we get stuck in old religious and medical maps that don't work and in many ways have caused a barrier to healing.

This book will not be embraced by the blamer simply because of the lack of appreciation for all things being purposeful. The person wanting to argue that sick is bad and healthy is good is stuck on judgment and separation. The person who wants to find an exception with genetics or an accident does the same.

For the same reasons you can't force someone into loving you with fear, coercion, money, or guilt – *The focus is the outcome.*

If the focus is based upon good or bad, fear or guilt, then the outcome will be built upon the same foundation of that focus.

It is why addiction programs and diets don't work. Without the shift from 'good' and 'bad', addiction, diet, illness and the like are stuck in a map that is perpetual. If we make the *focus* connecting with a higher purpose... the *outcome* is connecting with a higher purpose and true healing.

Money problems labeled as "bad" will automatically change the focus on whom or what is to blame. It is why 80 percent of people get stuck with money problems.

Relationship counselling that labels one or both partner's behavior as "bad' will always lead to two victims and two perpetrators in the relationship.

Health labeled as "bad" will lead you to focus on finding fault: which bug, which gene, which allergy, which food caused the problem...

Refer back to Newton's third law and the physics of change section for review while considering your references on things being good versus bad. For most people it is the television that invites guests into our home who teach and influence us. The TV shows, movies and news we watch focus almost entirely on "good" and "bad" versus looking at purpose and cause and effect. This makes it difficult to understand and embrace this map. What about religion and school? The undoing of the "bad" - "external" that causes blame and illness stops when we make the step towards things just being what they are. Either bringing us peace and our Grand Purpose or bringing to us that purposeful pain which tells us we are not at peace.

STEP 2: THOUGHTS, BELIEFS, FEELINGS, JUDGMENTS & PROJECTIONS

"do not judge, or you too will be judged. For in the same way you judge others, you will be judged, and with the measure you use, it will be measured to you." (Matthew 7:1-2)

This section is the big shift—the inertia that pushes us from external to internal. One of the key points is to understand that the judgments, projections, feelings, etc. are "descriptive." They are not external things as most have been taught. When something is descriptive it is internal. When these thoughts, beliefs, feelings, and projections are descriptive, internal manifestations, they easily become temporary and specific aspects of a changing you—the child of God that you are. By understanding this, change is no longer scary.

When I say descriptive, I am saying that our thoughts, beliefs, feelings, judgments and/or projections are simply describing an old me. If I say I am depressing, it is descriptive of a state that I am in versus "I am depressed" being an external 'thing'.

When someone says "I am not motivated," or "I am addicted," it is an external thing that is permanent and pervasive. When they shift to a descriptive explanation of motivating or addicting—we ask: What is motivation? What is addiction? Just like depression, we shift from unmotivated to "un-motivating." Just like depressing it is a non-tangible act of being. When you understand this—you own your destiny.

"Depressed" is not "real", nor is "motivation". Depressing and motivating are real; they are a state of mind. This linguistic difference is the start of making a change: our words we use, leading to our thoughts and feelings. The addiction to these feelings and thoughts is the sticking point. Take an unmotivated person and put a gun to their head and see how real this thing called motivation is.

The challenge is that this book does not explain every thought, belief, feeling, judgment and projection in terms of external versus internal. You're going to have to exercise your heart and brain. The "just like me" exercise below helps. Our eyes project outwards making it difficult or next to impossible to see ourselves. It is in relationships that we are able to see ourselves in who we see in the relationship. The workbook will address change through your own power. It will do so by seeing yourself through a different lens and using relationships as your compass. When a healthy person gives you feedback, use it to empower. Ask healthy people for their opinion on your shortcomings. Use the judgments and opinions of the unhealthy people in your life as a guide as well.

Just like me:

One of my favorite and most moving exercises is to use this simple quote whenever I am judging, believing, thinking and/or projecting. It's simple. If I say *that guy is an idiot*, I immediately say "just like me." It again makes it descriptive. What this does is flood me with feelings and insight about me feeling and thinking this way. The "just like me" exercise may temporarily be uncomfortable and messy; just focus on the fact that the mess will bring about wholeness. If I am in blame, I am in error... If I am in pain, I am in error.

To benefit from this book you must be open to the idea that illness starts in the mind. We all judge—some of us are conscious of it, some don't express their judgments and the outcome is the same. An internal insult to our own self is probably the single most impedance to healing. Judgments are purposeful as all illness is purposeful. They both give us feedback on where the cause is.

It does not matter if the judgment is about money, relationships or health. If you judge money as bad or scarce then that judgment sabotages. The same in relationships: If you judge your partner with the projections and limitations you impose on yourself you will have problems in your relationship. The adage that you have to love yourself to be able to love is solid. In health, judgments may involve worthiness of being healthy, the possibility of being healthy because you believe in genetics, or that you don't have the time or resources to be healthy.

Instead of getting overwhelmed by this, take simple steps to change your language and internalize judgments; this will take practice and most importantly, be gentle with yourself.

**Key Step: I am being _____ (feeling, judgment, projection, thought; i.e. depressing, angry...)

I feel grateful to experience feeling _____ (feeling, judgment, projection, thought; i.e. depressing, angry, control...)

HEALTH: IT IS WHERE IT ISN'T

We have come to appreciate a counterintuitive approach to solving many problems. Health's answers are also counterintuitive. We will not solve the high number of gun deaths in this country by focusing on the bullets. We will not solve health issues by focusing on diet and genetics. While bullets and nutrition do cause death, hopefully we can agree that they are not the cause. One of my biggest challenges in walking with people in their journey is changing the focus from fighting the condition to accepting it—then thanking it!

Someone comes to me with depression, thyroid problems, or arthritis... We do this workbook and suggest they do a water fast. The shift is to not make the fast about the condition. The reason the water fast is not combative is that it addresses the addiction by way of virtue, abstaining from the addictive source in an internal way which allows healing. The fast is about becoming whole, not losing weight or curing a condition. The simultaneous healing of the body and mind are absolute in the water fast if it is conducted from the internal.

ADDICTING AND SECONDARY GAINS
"...for my power is made perfect in weakness" Jesus

I usually explain this process by my explanation of shifting the person who believes in the disease called Depression (see step 1). Understanding that the following exercises are based on being empowered and calling yourself on these "off-nesses" brings you to your Grand Purpose. This is done by making the following difficult assertions temporary and specific, not getting crippled by making them permanent and pervasive. Once a person says "I am depressing" over and over again, it shifts to: This is temporary and specific. Ultimately it becomes fleeting and a thing of the past. The same applies to the following traps and the challenging patterns that cause illness.

To take a little emotion out of it we can take a step back and look at what happens to a child that is afraid of the boogeyman under his bed. Mom or dad come by the bedroom at 10 pm and see the light on. They say "Johnny it is a school night, you need to go to bed." Johnny says "But I am scared because I think there is something under the bed." Mom, fatigued and irritated at the thought of dealing with an exhausted Jonny the next morning says, "Don't be silly... don't be afraid, there is nothing under the bed." What just happened is the realness of Johnny's fear was turned off and stunted. We all know that there is no boogeyman and the child's wild imagination of hearing springs move in the bed create this real feeling of fear. Unless it is validated as real, and, importantly, allowed, this child will learn to suppress feelings. Not good. We need to allow the child to feel the fear then it goes away. "Johnny, I understand that you are fearful, most kids feel this way because of the noises and being in the dark alone..."

The same applies to telling Jonny that he did great at soccer when he is terrible or mediocre. These "benign" optimistic lies encourage lying to ourselves. It creates subconscious, pessimistic views. This leads to misguided optimism and pessimism with medical conditions, finances, and relationship problems. These exercises are the balance needed to create change... It is where the rubber meets the road.

COMMON FOCUS
& HOW TO CORRECT THEM

Blaming on external luck, chance or genetics does not bring resolve. More than half of the millionaires in the world have gone bankrupt. The key distinction between those who stay in financial crisis versus those who heal is that the person consciously or subconsciously admits to being lazy, greedy, etc. When The Grand Purpose is adopted it makes it easy to be gentle, confess and be humble. Money, relationship and health problems are commonly rooted in the following:

> Money: greed, entitlement, temptation, laziness, envy, indulgence
> Relationships: insecure, hostile
> Health: laziness, temptation, indulgence (see below)

THE EMOTIONAL BAGGAGE
"We sink to rise" Ralph Waldo Emerson

The Victim is the Perpetrator: How radical but true! If you do the work in this workbook, you will realize that there is no difference between the victim and perpetrator except what we have been brainwashed into thinking: One is bad and one is noble. This is a gentle, non-judgmental approach to changing and healing by looking internal for the victim. Remember the virus (perp) only takes on the host (victim) if there is a suitable environment. Note: we are not claiming that the victim is bad, evil, guilty or at fault.

Studies have shown that victims give off a certain level of victimness. Perpetrators, when asked why they chose this person versus that person, will give subjective answers as to why, by stating that one person "feels" like a victim and another doesn't. *That person will fight back, that person won't.*

When I talk openly with the victims, the honesty is compelling. Those who have been a victim and sought refuge with the courts—and the jury that feels sorry for them—realize they are not getting their needs met and must change themselves to escape the trap. Others become addicted to being a victim and seek any person to listen to their story while alienating all healthy people. For those who come to the conclusion that getting mugged is a form of getting touched, or heard or seen, Wow! What an *ah-ha* moment. They heal and change; they realize that they are looking for love in the wrong place and they must change internally to find real love… It is truly a humbling and liberating moment.

One healthy way to address being a "victim" is to say: Yes, I have been wrong, that's okay. If it keeps happening it's probably me. Another outlook is to say: "Yes, I have been wrong, that's okay. What can I do about it?"

"Have no friend not equal to yourself" —Confucius

I have had the same insightful dialogue with many women struggling with thyroid and weight problems that discuss their history of sexual abuse. What is again humbling and healing is watching these women gently take control by internalizing the event: seeking what it was they were needing when it happened. They no longer need to blame the uncle (virus), ex-husband (bacteria), etc. They have no need to be a victim; how quickly the guilt, humiliation, and shame melt away. The only regret, why didn't I do this years ago?

Let's back up one more step and agree that all perpetrators have suffered being the victim of abuse or mistrust at some point in the past. Instead of surrendering to being a victim themselves or retreating and avoiding relationships they swing the pendulum in the opposite direction and *get others* before they get them. All perpetrators have been the victim. In conclusion, we agree that the victim turned into the perpetrator. The next leap is that any person not exposed to abuse or mistrust would not attract such negative behavior.

Now let's look at the victim of abuse or mistrust that, instead of swinging the pendulum, subconsciously seeks abuse to validate the learned behavior. Are they somehow to blame? I suggest no, and at the same time we need to ask the same germ theory questions we ask about the virus and the healthy person. Psychology or social work does not have a resolution for this dance. It blames the perpetrator and feels sorry for the victim.

If the perpetrator is the virus and the victim is the person catching the virus, we must ask why the perpetrator could not take a hold of the healthy person. In the new Map or Grand Purpose model, we don't blame the virus. We thank it for bringing us the awareness that we are off. It is a perfect analogy.

Are we going to blame the person getting raped for asking for it? No. In my experience of people healing, the common denominator is the person who was raped coming to terms that on some level they needed or attracted it and no longer need that kind of negative reinforcement to get love or attention. The result is healing. The stark difference to many people's knee-jerk reaction upon reading this is that of blame, shame, and guilt. These feelings are a result of using the wrong map.

We go back to the 'just like me' exercise: *I feel abused when you hit me*, or *I feel abused when you call me names*. The Grand Purpose approach: *I am being abusing...* which leads ultimately to: *I have no need in my life for abuse*. This progression and healing takes work and the ability to get a little messy in the process.

Only when the victim can own their passive-aggressiveness as a violent form of abuse can they heal. Passive aggressiveness has become art in the victim's broken record. Other times victims are not passive aggressive and just blaming other external factors. Either way, the path to healing occurs when we internalize and be gentle with ourselves.

Don't blame the attacker; even though most therapists will tell you that you should or can. Blame sounds like this: "But I was only eight years old..." The truth is you cannot change or reform the attacker, so your emotions are futile. No man can save his brother's soul or pay his brother's debt. The truth is you cannot "fix" anyone, nor do they require your "fixing." You can only work on yourself. So often people get caught up in the incomplete paradigm of blaming the people in their lives, that they miss the need to change and heal within themselves.

After entering this new-map approach of internalizing in a gentle way you can see that it all follows common sense.

This same approach applies to giving and receiving, controlling and being controlled, being critical and criticizing. You can't have one without the other. If you have trouble receiving because you self-sacrifice herein lies your challenge. If being controlled by someone is an issue then look at your need to be controlled as a passive-aggressive way of controlling. If you are hypercritical of others or situations, is it possible that you are harsh or critical of yourself?

It is easy to see that mean, pretty girls need to insult the other girls because in doing so the insult temporarily boosts the pretty girl's low self-esteem giving her a high that is short-lived. Does this go both ways?

If we simply put these patterns of dysfunction in an internal framework of internal descriptive dialogue, change happens always. The Grand Purpose of a Condition: From Head To Toe (See The Course In Health Workbook).

"Everything is connected... no one thing can change by itself." Paul Hawken

Simply put each organ, limb, and system of our body has a purpose. Some are very obvious, others are less. This became validated when in the 1980's medical doctors and the media became vocal when they connected ulcers in the stomach to the emotion of worry. This awareness became accepted medical advice and the incidence of ulcers decreased tremendously. The obvious reason was the awareness of the emotional link. When worried people felt worry, their awareness prevented them from holding the emotion in their stomach, thus preventing the ulcer. Nowadays, since most people have not heard this from their well-respected doctor, ulcers are coming back. The mainstream medical approach has started to prove the same with medical studies showing the connection between emotions and certain cancers, heart disease and diabetes.

EFFECT TO CAUSE -
A MESSY CONNECTION

Those stuck on the germ theory have a difficult time with the following process. This "Map" process is focused on painful feelings or personality traits being temporary and specific. It is however very personal and messy for some. These realizations or conclusions from effect to cause are many years of clinical results that people have resolved; I was just there facilitating.

When an authentic, good-hearted woman who is overweight uses physics to resolve her conflict with the abuse that was closer to the root of needing to gain weight, the results become lasting and healing.

Pain is purposeful. Emotions serve a purpose. Either the emotion is bringing us toward our Grand Purpose, or it is missing the mark. Emotions that miss the mark are addressed below.

Remember messy is not "bad." The messy kitchen that is required to make a great meal is necessary, and those labeling the mess as bad may not get to eat.

STEP 3 - BREATHE

Master your breath, Master your mind. In the year 1990 I took yoga breathing classes in Vancouver British Columbia. The science and eastern philosophy of this training has not changed in all these years and for 20 years in practice I have provided breathing instruction to patients as a part of the foundation to health. Keep these exercises simple, as they are intended to be.

The first thing we do when we are born is take a breath; when we die we expire. Throughout life we require the cycle of respiration to maintain our existence.

The cycle of digestion of food takes twenty-four hours.

The cycle of respiration, or digestion of air, takes approximately three seconds.

We can live without food for approximately 40 days.

We can live without water for about four days.

We can live without air for about four minutes.

Even with the clear physiological necessity ofthe breath, there is even a more marvelous and spectacular aspect of the breath. It is the fact that it is one of the only things that connects our minds with our bodies. With each breath comes a new thought or expression of life.

A basic understanding of the parasympathetic and the sympathetic nervous systems highlights the magnificence of the breath. The sympathetic nervous system is our fight-or-flight system consisting of activities related to the gas pedal, and the parasympathetic system is our rest-and-digest, or the brake pedal of our nervous system.

PARASYMPATHETIC	SYMPATHETIC
• Constricts pupils	Dilated pupil
• Increase saliva	Decrease saliva
• Decrease heart rate	Increase heart rate
• Constricts bronchial airway	Dilates bronchial airway
• Stimulates digestion	Inhibits digestion
• Constricts bladder	Dilates bladder
• Stimulates sexual arousal	Stimulates orgasm

Both systems control the function of digestive, cardiovascular, and hormonal for our organs and systems. The overall system governing the parasympathetic and sympathetic is the autonomic nervous system, synonymous with autonomic nervous system. We don't have to tell our heart to beat or our kidneys to filter blood or tell our stomach to create digestive enzymes. All systems are controlled by the autonomic nervous system. For example, the heart, when it needs to beat fast, utilizes the sympathetic system and slows down the parasympathetic system. We don't have to consciously ask our central nervous system to beat our heart, it just does so automatically. Of all the functions and systems we do have control over it is our breath and the blinking and closing of our eyes. We can slow down or speed up our breathing by way of thought. This is profound, and I will get back to this.

Our breathing can then be both conscious and unconscious. When we sleep—or are not thinking about breathing—it is unconscious, automatic or non-volitional.

By this very fact, the breath becomes the connection between the mind and the body, or the yin and the yang, between the masculine and the feminine.

Through alternate nostril breathing we are able to connect the polarity of the brain to encourage balance and healing. As written, healing is said to occur when the left brain connects with the right brain; when the masculine and feminine connect to become whole. Breathing is the transformative tool to connect us.

An understanding of the fact that humans are electromagnetic beings reduced to a cup full of ash upon death, what gives us life force is the fact that we are electromagnetic beings. Where this electromagnetic component comes from is our cerebrospinal fluid. The connection between our cerebrospinal fluid and our breathing is a direct one. We have something called a cranial sacral respiratory system in which the cranium and the sacrum move together to pump and ionize the cerebrospinal fluid. Breathing is the catalyst to this function by pumping this fluid throughout our central nervous system

Abdominal breathing is the most natural and fluid act of a healthy newborn baby: the little belly extending and filling the lungs with life force in every pump. When the belly extends and the diaphragm relaxes it causes a vacuum of air to fill the entire lung: the abdominal muscles relaxing and diaphragm contracting with exhalation naturally forcing air out with vacuum pressure. It is efficient. This process repeats itself until some stress or interference causes the breath to be altered. The child being yelled at or alarmed creates the parasympathetic system to shift to the sympathetic and the breath becomes short and shallow consistent with the fight or flight. The baby transitions to chest breathing. There is physiological and survival purpose in sympathetic breathing. Short, rapid and shallow chest breathing allows the fight or flight. It is to preserve life throughout life.

It is when the stress goes away and the breathing has not restored to abdominal do we start to see problems. In the adult, with ailments or addictions, we see chest breathing (sympathetic). In the chronic sympathetic state, we do not see the balance that is required to heal and illness progresses. This often progresses to mouth breathing.

Without abdominal breathing we do not access the cranial sacral respiratory motion, the abdominal movement does not positively move and exercise the organs, and the cerebrospinal fluid does not get the conductor of energy required to maximize life. Within our nostrils, we have cranial nerves that are the only nerves with direct access to our brains. When we breathe in and out of the nostrils we ionize the air, giving it an electrical charge to help start the efficient energy cycle.

When breathing is not balanced, it will affect our sleep patterns. Understand that our sympathetic nervous system should take a rest during sleep and the parasympathetic system (rest and digest) takes charge. When sleep is disturbed we are unable to process life events, eliminate toxins, etc.

Understanding how important it is to have parasympathetic dominance during rest and digestion is key. When we eat we must be relaxed. In doing so, our bodies can secrete parasympathetic digestive enzymes to break down food. If we are in the sympathetic state it is not possible, and digestion suffers (heartburn, acid reflux, etc.).

When breathing is not balanced and relaxed it has a direct effect on our nervous system. Alternate nostril breathing exercises are the quickest way to restore balance.

We have nostril dominance that changes throughout the day. If you check your nostril dominance now you will have one that is partially blocked and one fully open. In a healthy person, this dominance changes every few hours. This physiological gift allows the body to ionize both hemispheres of the brain to allow healing. When people are stressed or unhealthy, the nostril dominance does not shift or shifts less frequently. The nostril breathing exercise encourages the rebalancing to occur.

A change in the physical body starts with the holding of the breath and the negative thoughts. We hold onto the thought and it manifests into a physical ailment, muscle tension, or postural change. If illness starts in the mind and the breath is connected to the mind, it is a logical starting point.

Proper control of your breath is the secret to manifesting self-control and self-awareness. It is impossible to be in a parasympathetic state and experience negative emotions or a vice.

Breathing Exercises: Refer to Website instruction video

All four breathing exercises are performed daily and are through the nostrils (both inhalation and exhalation). Ratios for Abdominal Breathing and Alternate Nostril Breathing:

Start with a 1:2 ratio - Inhalation (1): Exhalation (2)

For example, start with inhalation for three seconds and exhalation for six. Progress to 4:8 and when 4:8 is comfortable to proceed to the next ratio.

Begin these exercises with the ratio of '3 sec: 12 sec: 6 sec.' This is 'inhalation: hold: exhalation.' You will gradually increase your lung capacity and therefore increase the numbers in the ratio. This increase will come with time and the regularity of the exercises performed. Make sure you are 100 percent comfortable with the current ratio you are using before increasing to the next ratio. I advise practicing these techniques first thing in the morning or afternoon. Doing them before bedtime may interfere with sleep.

1. Abdominal Breathing - 3 minutes

Minimum of 4 minutes a day. It is a good idea to do these exercises twice a day for the first two weeks.

Lay on a firm surface (floor). No pillow.

Concentrate on expanding your chest with each breath in (push your stomach out like a "pregnant belly" to make room for your diaphragm to descend while inhaling). Concentrate on sucking your belly in with each breath out to push your diaphragm back up. Remember, no movement in the ribs. Remember to inhale and exhale through the nose.

2. Alternate Nostril Breathing: 3 minutes

Using your thumb to depress one nostril, inhale for three seconds, then hold (index finger is placed gently between brows on your forehead for stabilization). While holding your breath a total of 12 seconds, release nostril and depress opposite nostril with your middle finger, and continue holding then exhale for six counts. Without changing fingers, inhale for three, hold 12, then change nostrils and exhale for six. One rep is in-out-in-out. Do five reps to make one set. Do one to five sets. Use the same ratio as the abdominal breathing.

3. Shoulder Breathing: 1- 3 minutes

Inhale, raise shoulders as far as you can towards the ears. Exhale quickly and drop shoulders completely. Done correctly, you will experience a small bounce in your shoulders when you release. The ratio for this exercise is just 1:1.

4. Quiet Lying Breathing: 1 - 2 minutes

Lying on your back, breathing through your nose, allow your mind to escape. If stress or daily thoughts keep rising, count down from 100 (i.e. 100, 99, 98, 97, ...). If you lose concentration start over.

STEP 4 - VISUALIZATION

"For everyone who asks receives, and he who seeks finds, and to him who knocks it will be opened." (Matthew 7:8)

Visualization starts with the end in mind. It only asks for what is real—to accept what was already given. See it—then you will be it. This is the simplest exercise to understand your limitation on belief in that if you can't see it you don't believe it. Decide what you want (not what you don't want) and create a clear picture of it until it gets so clear you can feel it and see it.

When the picture is difficult to see it simply guides us back to step one and two.

This exercise is not to make "bad" things go away. Ignore the things you think you need; instead focus on your <u>purpose</u>.

Visualize – Details of work/profession that energizes you

Visualize – Details of financial well-being

Visualize – Details of where and when you would travel

Visualize – Exercises that you love to do: the excitement, joy, peace

Visualize – Details of your level of energy

Visualize – Your ideal body and self-image

Visualize – Your relationships – communication, affection. New ones, mended ones, maintained

Visualize – Your special interests or hobbies

Keep it simple: close your eyes and visualize until you see it. It does take practice. If you struggle, start with easy visualizations. Visualize present and future.

Pray and Meditate with an internal focus. Ask for nothing; just focus on your Grand Purpose. Don't focus on needs, only on purpose and your truth and gratitude through forgiveness.

The commitment is to be honest with your thoughts—with the openness of changing your consciousness—by changing these thoughts through these first four steps.

EXERCISE - SELF-CONTROL SELF-AWARENESS

Do you ever watch people who exhibit great self-control? They eat until they are full and don't overeat. They don't overspend and they stop at one glass of wine. They don't gossip. They exercise without needing a trainer or coach. It's not magic. First secret is relationships: positive, healthy people around them, role models or mentors, honest and caring critics, etc.

The secret is expanding on what it is you value or what your purpose is in life. When you have a powerful *why*, the *how* comes with ease and self-control.

EXERCISE - VALUES EXERCISE

Who are you? What are your gifts, strengths or abilities? What is the meaning of your life? What is your purpose? What are your goals? How do you want to be remembered? Why do you do your daily duties? What makes you tick? How do you make decisions?

These are crucial questions that most Americans have not addressed. Because of this lack of clarity, we see people struggle when trying to make choices that are consistent with growth or healing. Once the exercises are completed, however, there is room for congruency in our daily lives. We are able to identify what is important and act upon it. Most people say they value health, but when we look at their behavior, we wonder. Their actions very often reveal their dilemma. For example, eating McDonald's or other fast food twice a week, drinking sodas, not exercising, or not getting enough sleep are indicative of a dilemma. We can apply this question to anything we say we value. Valuing family, for instance, cannot include such habits as working 60 plus hours a week, coming home too exhausted to do anything, and sprawling before the television. These behaviors must then be rationalized or compartmentalized, but this will not prevent the trauma to the psyche, which recognizes the dilemma, and resents it. Recognizing your inconsistencies will open the door to alternative choices. Again, we see the power of creating a "why" so that the "how" becomes easy. The powerful "whys" are your values. For example, a mother who instinctively values the needs of her newborn will find it relatively easy to get up several times each night.

There are no correct answers to values clarification. However, failing to complete this exercise (See The Course In Health Workbook for exercise) will prolong your growth, deter your healing and you will remain a stranger to the most important person in your life – You.

The key to this exercise is to spend quality time asking yourself these questions, and reflecting upon your answers. Write them down. Once you have done that, look at them to evaluate how your daily activities relate to what you value.

Once you have completed this exercise, congratulate yourself. You have just identified your priorities in life. These values or priorities will help and guide you through decisions of the future. The next step is to learn ways to act upon your newly established priorities. Obviously the list is not complete, but it will get you started. Feel free to make your own additions. From the list below choose words that hold meaning in your life. You may choose as many or as few as you desire.

Doing this exercisedoesn't mean that you will make all the "correct" choices. It simply allows you to see where your actions are consistent with your values. When our actions are not consistent, we can be pretty certain that we have some limiting beliefs and/or patterns at work in our lives.

A tool that has had a tremendous effect in accessing these values is verbalizing the truth of your actions. For example, if I work long hours I say, "Right now, work is more important than being with my son, or relaxing."

EXERCISE - JOURNAL

Your words—questions/thoughts—will always produce your reality. This is fact. The scientific explanation is simple: Your thoughts are things. These "things" are therefore "real" (as far as our physical reality). The analogy is: if a bullet from a gun is real, it is a thing; it would be safe to say that this bullet can do harm, just as a thought. On the other hand if the thought is:'loving' (the true meaning of real) it will produce peace. Remember it all starts with your words.

THE *FASTEST* WAY TO RECOVERY

When addiction or any illness is an issue, I have found water fasting is the most profound way to heal. This addresses the addiction without shifting from one addiction to another. If your addiction is gambling, food, high blood pressure, obesity or any addiction... consider therapeutic fasting. The physiological and emotional benefits are simultaneous. The dualistic effect of the fast is one of the most remarkable aspects. Doctors who supervise therapeutic fasting have the ability to address the deep emotional change that results during the fast (something that does not happen when getting treated with natural or synthetic pills of other treatments).

Some patients believe that their knowledgeable doctor directing them on the length of the fast or monitoring their vitals and lab work is the most critical aspect of the fast. However, doctors would agree that the most profound aspect of the fast is the driver of the fast: the customer. They are doing all the work and require all the credit. Doctors observing or guiding and/or studying the customer would agree that the single biggest hurdle in dealing with the person fasting is their emotional state. Often the person wants to stop the fast due to emotional discomfort.

If you have done a water fast and not received lasting results please reconsider your focus and Grand Purpose in doing the fast. Do the fast after completing the steps in the workbook and make the fast only about your Grand Purpose, not about fighting a condition.

I have been recommending fasting for 20 plus years. I have always believed fasting to be the ideal path to health from mild to complicated medical issues. While I believe any person can navigate a fast successfully I have also received a steady flow of phone calls from people doing fasts on their own, calling me in desperation. The most common key to failure in the fasting process by the doctor and/or the patient is their attempt to treat the "disease"—chasing your health from outside. This workbook has hopefully guided you to look inward: What if…

What if we do what we do for one Grand Purpose? What if we don't know our Grand Purpose and what we do creates pain? What if the pain is intended to guide you to your Grand Purpose? That Grand Purpose is your quest; it may be to find a higher purpose, love, unity, or God. In that quest for your Grand Purpose, we use maps given to us. Some maps are ineffective—they are traps. If the map you choose is correct, you heal.

A demonstration is the single most determination of what is real. Don't confuse this with testimonials. Fasting is healing each and every time. I know that these steps offer the demonstration that allows fasting to create a permanent change of consciousness when the focus is internal.

In the movie, Talladega Nights, Ricky Bobby is quoted as saying: "You gotta win to get love, everybody knows it; it's just the way it is." The irony and pain in this statement is what I believe is in all addictions and all illness. We do what we do to become whole. When fear, worry, anger or any vice interferes with that attempt to be whole, we resort to behaviors/actions that will subconsciously get us love. For some that may be getting sick to get love, for others it may be an addiction to perfectionism to get love, others may hit rock bottom with drugs or alcohol to have their love met. If you don't believe we get sick for emotional reasons, talk to those who have healed, or talk to those overcoming addiction—thanking every part of it. Only through a change of consciousness do we heal. The late H.H. "Doc" Robertson, a great doctor and teacher, taught me that there are no incurable conditions—only incurable people. This workbook allows you to change your consciousness on your terms.

TRAUMA OR ACCIDENTS OR BEING A VICTIM?

Trauma or accident is the result of many factors. For example, trauma can be overexposure to dangerous situations or a weakened ligament in your shoulder which finally gives way when you toss a ball. Calcium, magnesium and essential fatty acid deficiency will eventually weaken bone mass, which leaves one more susceptible to fractures. Manganese deficiency can produce weakness in the spinal discs, leaving one vulnerable to back pain due to herniated discs. Excess pyruvic and lactic acid from an excess of carbohydrates in the diet, along with a deficiency of vitamin B6 can lead to carpal tunnel syndrome, sciatica, and other neuralgia-like pain. I could go on and on. When someone performs a task hundreds of times with no trauma, then suddenly the task causes trauma, it is fair to conclude that it is likely the weakened structure and not the trauma. However, we are taught to blame or focus on the trauma or accident.

As I have pointed out throughout this book, the primary cause is emotional. There are no exceptions. The next question I often hear is, "What about car accidents, or trauma as a result of someone or something beyond my direct control?" Once again, I can only say, there are no accidents. There are subconscious factors at play. You put yourself in this situation. It is leading you to something you need to learn at exactly this point in your life. *"And we know that in all things God works for the good of those who love him..."* (Romans 8:28)

I presented this concept to a patient, just as I present it to all new patients. I was expecting debate and resistance as usual. This time, however, the patient volunteered that she understood her accident was part of her destiny. She was a passenger, yet she accepted responsibility for the accident! She went on to say that the driver had not been careless. The attorneys urged her to think of something, anything, which she could pin on the driver (blame). She would not. As a result, with every excuse in the book available to her, she took full responsibility for the back pain she is now experiencing. This woman had been doing her spiritual work and had expressed her willingness to accept better answers for her peace.

The same process has led other patients to accept this when "accidents" have occurred in their lives. In retrospect, many people subconsciously get sick or get in an accident because it fills their life with some distorted purpose. If someone is bored or has no purpose or goals, getting sick can fill the void. Quote by Albert Einstein: *"If you cause an accident, then it is not an accident."* Look deeper, and you will realize that even if you were not the one to go through the red light, you are still the cause of the accident because you were there. Some have linked accidents to a rebellion against authority or just anger. I love to go on long hikes in the mountains—sometimes 20 plus miles in a day. The times when I or a companion have tripped (no accident) and fallen I immediately ask myself what was my thought at that moment. Amazingly it was always some negative thought, anger, frustration. Then bang! A whisper through the fall. An old hiking friend Brian is the person that pointed this out to me of which I have shared with friends while hiking. If we don't immediately link the emotion with the action, it is often fleeting.

In talking to some of my friends that employ construction workers, there is a unanimous opinion that only those who "don't want to work" get injured at work. When you understand the Emotion Link and appreciate how many people are unhappy with their work it is an easy conclusion.

Victim: A person harmed (i.e. in a crime, accident, ordisaster) or a person harmed by an action or circumstance, or simply duped or tricked or exploited. The victim role falls within the previous section of accidents. "It wasn't my fault...This person did me wrong and was found guilty..." A careful look at this reveals physiological profiles of the victims that attract these events. Most people can relate to observing people who attract relationships that are abusive (sexual, physical or emotional) and repeat the dance with someone new after the old has dissolved; the same experience with a different mate. Is something compelling this person to be attracted to this type of person? Is there a reason for this relationship to manifest? Will this person attract different personality traits if they adopt the complete paradigm and look *within* rather than blame? Like attracts like—the mirror reflects back what is projected at it. Someone who has issues with trust or abuse will attract someone with those issues; opposites do not attract. The virus is attracted to the swamp. Sometimes someone who surrenders to abuse thinks subconsciously that they deserve to be punished and will attract someone who overcompensates by getting others before someone gets them. The subconscious goal is to attract someone who is uniquely unqualified to provide to you what you need to heal. This purposefully opens the wound to allow resolve through and by conflict or pain. Most relationships do not need extreme labels of victim and perpetrator. For explanation we can use the extreme by addressing the victim or the perpetrator: the "viruses" and the swamp. The virus seeks out those who are a suitable environment to thrive. For the victim they subconsciously seek or have the suitable environment for the perpetrator to act upon them.

In the workbook, we go into full detail concerning the victim-perpetrator connection and subsequent healing.

Fault, Blame, and Guilt. An explanation why fault, blame, and guilt are never used in this book to address healing is necessary. These focuses are linked to the external causes of the disease being luck, chance or genetics. Changing from luck, chance or genetics to fault, blame or guilt is a way to subconsciously avoid going internal.

Often I will have a patient question me by stating: "You're not telling me that the person getting hit by a drunk driver is at fault" or "You're not telling me that a kid who has a genetic condition is to blame."

The reason it is not possible to answer a question that assumes conclusions which are not concluded is that nowhere in this book does fault, blame, and guilt get linked to illness. Those words are a different map from a different planet. Healing uses internal framework set out in this book.

As you can see the virus or bug is not the fault, blame, or guilt causing the illness. The internal framework does not blame a virus that is opportunistic and purposeful in your health and healing.

The God I believe in responds to the internal that is forgiving, loving, virtuous and purposeful—not fault, blame, or guilt.

Fault, blame, and guilt assume that the virus is the enemy. If it is not the enemy it is not to blame, nor is it guilty. I have come to believe that when my Grand Purpose or The Holy Spirit resides in me my life is internally-driven and peaceful. When I am separate from the Grand Purpose or the Holy Spirit then fault, blame, and guilt are my natural defenses and become the focus.

RELIGION IN HEALTHCARE

Many religions have rules and guidelines with respect to medical care. Seventh-day Adventist, the Buddhist Guidelines, Hindu Religion, Christian Science, Jehovah's Witness and other religions have logical beliefs that support healing without drugs and medical intervention.

It is not a coincidence that all religions have direction on addictive behavior; deterring those to abstain from alcohol, drugs, and gambling. The interesting leap is that all these religions have fasting as a practice. The connection is that practicing a religious fast requires virtue. Those addicted to food or drug must fast to heal from the vice.

Fasting, I believe, brings us very close to a raw state thus enables us to touch healing. Through fasting, most will realize that they are addicted to food. Being addicted to alcohol, painkillers, and gambling are more obvious. What makes the fast special is that link to a Grand Purpose through religion. The challenge for my therapeutic fasting practice is the focus of the fast being for weight loss, arthritis, cancer or blood pressure symptoms to go away. When the focus of the fast is external, like a treatment, pill or magic, many people do not get lasting results. When the focus is on a Grand Purpose or virtues we see lasting healing.

OUTSIDE - IN

At this point, let's agree that we have been looking for health in all the wrong places. We agree that the majority of natural and mainstream medical treatments are not addressing the factors causing illness. We agree that our healthcare system is unscientific. It leaves us with the question... what's next? First, we need to identify the cause of your condition, and then make the change.

Changing is relatively easy yet so evasive for many. Let's look and think outside the box about changing a behavior in a sport or hobby. Either trial and error or getting a lesson from someone who identifies a problem and shows an alternative successful approach, are ways to change and improve.

Changing a behavior/addiction happens all the time. The caution is not just stopping the addiction and substituting for another addiction… it's about making it last. Stopping problem-drinking just to substitute with cigarettes or food is not what I consider change.

Changing our personalities seems to be the greatest challenge. I believe that adopting virtues and changing significant personality flaws, tendencies or patterns is crucial in making the step to health.

Change happens when we either see a need to change or are forced to change. Any person with dilemmas or dis-ease in any area of their life has an opportunity to change. Those who are afraid of their potential will forever resist change. Those looking for a better way will start to embrace their opportunity.

Willingness to change usually goes hand in hand with hitting rock bottom. Humans always want a state that produces happiness, tending to move away from pain or toward pleasure. I believe that most of us live our lives seeking to avoid pain by making decisions based on fear. This pattern will change once you complete the values clarification exercise and your mission statement in the workbook, *and* find your purpose.

As explained earlier, our physical habits are merely a manifestation of our emotional habits. Our addiction behavior to a negative focus, or addictive, un-resourceful self-talk, has in the past served a purpose. Your job in your self-assessment is to find out the *purpose* it served in order to *resolve* the emotion involved. The ability to change our physical behaviors has to do with the speed at which a physical act is conducted. For example, the time it takes to reach for a donut or coke is relatively long, and we can easily stop in mid-motion. When we look at addictive thoughts that are not serving us, the process is far too rapid for interjection. To change thoughts we must change habits in advance, and purposefully.

SECTION 9

PHYSICS AND CHANGE

Newton's third law: Every action has an opposite and equal reaction. Is change difficult or easy? Change is neither easy nor difficult; it is relative to a person's perception or thoughts regarding the result of the change and most importantly their Grand Purpose, values, and goals. When someone clarifies their values and is 'on purpose,' change is a smooth transition.

If your goal is to cease to engage in destructive behavior, thought, or food, etc., and you crave or can't stop the behavior, relax and do not force the change. Physics is vital to change. For example, take eating potato chips: We have concluded that hydrogenated oils (potato chips) cause many symptoms and illnesses. For you, it might be headaches or a skin problem. Your doctor has empowered you with this education, you feel better when you don't eat these toxic foods, but for whatever reason, you continue to eat them even though they are toxic.

The key to making change resides in your internal questions, dialogue/thoughts, and values clarification. "The real seat of taste was not the tongue but the mind," and comes with the will, wisdom, and power to change (Gandhi).

Exercise: Say, "I am a good person for wanting to change. Eating this food (or substitute with behavior) does not bring me closer to my Grand Purpose in loving and respecting myself."

When the refined sugar or alcohol is causing problems in your life and your well-intentioned doctor tells you to stop eating sugar or stop drinking alcohol... a very, very small percentage of people are successful at lasting change. When someone tells you what you are doing is bad or wrong and that 'something' brings you great pleasure your brain gets confused; it creates a dilemma. The dilemma is you want to be healthy but you don't want to give up what gives you pleasure. When you see the donut or glass of wine, your craving is physiologic. Because you want "health" you choose to have willpower and abstain from the donut. Then after several weeks (the most 6 months) the willpower is overtaken by your subconscious addiction and connection with the donut. You see the donut and you start to rationalize that eating only one donut will do no harm and eating things in moderation is the way to go. Unfortunately the side effect with this compartmentalization is that you associate failure, shame and/or guilt with eating the donut, which also produces pain in your brain. Because this conflict is so stressful, you (subconsciously) need to pick one side. You then subconsciously decide that the pain of giving up the donut is too great, and you associate more pain with being a failure and you then subconsciously decide that being healthy is too difficult. Therefore, you associate pain with the diet and ultimately gain more weight than before. One way to make these changes last is to be gentle on yourself when wanting to eliminate the "donut" from your life. Tell yourself that the donut causes pain and the broccoli creates pleasure. The process is similar: you commit to making a change—the difference is you are not associating failure, shame or guilt with the donut—you associate pain instead. So when you tell yourself that donuts cause ill health or weight gain the choice not to eat them becomes an internal focus and you associate pleasure with staying away. Then the emotional trigger kicks in several months down the road. Instead of making excuses for why you are eating the donut you instead tell yourself gently: "This donut does not bring me closer to my goals, it brings me further. This particular time I choose the short term pleasure the donut gives me over the long-term costs." What happens is honest and impressionable to your subconscious. The dilemma is confronted. Now the subconscious weighs the cost and benefits and does not have failure, guilt or shame clouding its path. At some point, after eating donuts you start to associate distaste and pain when you eat one. You essentially change your taste for the donuts from a place of pleasure to disgust. This is how purpose and virtues are attained. As Gandhi has stated, "The real seat of taste was not the tongue but the mind."

When this happens, the donut tastes terrible, and you have evolved/changed to desire something healthier for yourself. It is a profound experience to truly change your experience and sensation of something addictive by internalizing your perceptions and connecting them to purpose. When this happens, you can now change your focus on the emotional trigger that leads to the craving of the donut. When I think about this event I crave the donut. We then see the purpose of craving the donut. The craving of the donut is to help deflect the pain of the negative experience. The donut and the chemicals change brain chemistry to numb the pain temporarily. The problem is the negative side effects of the junk food. When we start to identify with the emotional trigger, we can then take a more productive approach to these triggers and use tools that allow us to resolve these emotional issues that don't involve food, drugs, internet, etc.

This ties into all addictions and change. The person who uses drugs or alcohol to escape from emotional issues is no different than the person eating donuts, or the person using the internet, or work, etc. Addictions and these behaviors are coping mechanisms to avoid the pain. The healthy person who is confronted with an emotional issue chooses to address the issue with one or several healthy coping tools like expressing their feelings, talking, exercising, praying, forgiving, breathing, etc. When the resolution is reached, there is no need to cover up the pain with addictions because there is no pain to cover up. Our medical system, schools, and parents often do not teach healthy coping skills and instead teach us to use pills or blame for emotional hurts that lead to covering up the pain. Simply put, the person using alcohol to numb the pain is doing so because that is what he knows helps get rid of the pain. KEY POINT: If you are in pain, your brain tells you to get out of it because pain is stressful to our bodies and mind. If your brain does not direct you to natural healthy ways to get rid of the pain your brain is perfectly okay with toxic ways to get rid of the pain. It is well-established that drugs and alcohol are excellent pain relievers with toxic side effects. They are superficial bandages. The drugs or alcohol are just buying time at a cost. They are allowing you to not address the emotional issue. Remember pain is purposeful: we need to ask what is the purpose and use it to guide us. Again I will use the money analogy. You have "money pain" and the band-aid for the money pain is to get a new credit card or get a loan. The credit is not addressing the money pain at its core. It temporarily makes the pain go away however the pain will come back if it is not addressed at the core.

The result is even more pain and more debt. The pain pills are high-interest cover-ups that cost you. It's okay to use them, just understand that there is a cost. Our financial system allows for fresh starts with bankruptcy; our physical bodies and relationships are not so forgiving. The bankruptcy equivalent in health is having a heart attack, getting diabetes or cancer, becoming obese, etc. In relationships, it's divorce.

Starting over can give a clean slate and become rewarding and spiritual for those who take responsibility. If we have learned and changed, we use these bankruptcies to make us whole, and we are thankful for the experience. We would not trade the circumstances because they lead us to peace. Because we move away from pain or towards pleasure the goal of healing is to shift from moving away from pain to moving towards pleasure (see The Course In Health Workbook).

THE FOCUS IS THE OUTCOME
IT'S NOT ALL OR NONE

An airplane in flight has a destination. While in flight the airplane is off course 90 percent of the time. The pilot continually makes slight corrections to put the plane back on path. The destination is therefore achieved, and no one seems to point out a more efficient manner of accomplishing this because there isn't one. You may not realize that driving a car is similar; the constant corrections you make in your steering keeps you on the course, and we don't complain about it. It has become second nature. We want the same focus to take hold in our health.

Your destination can be health, spirituality, relationships, love or whatever you truly value. Your means must adhere to the timeless principles described in this book. Embrace that you are continually getting off course and gently correct your behaviors and get to your destination. Remember the pilot and copilot are not yelling and blaming each other for being off 90 percent of the time. It is a gentle, objective dialogue. Often the getting off course is met with resistance, blame, denial, etc. This leads to stress that pushes people to take pills.

Going back to the airplane analogy and getting off course: blaming or denial never gets us to the destination. Just think about the pilots using blame or denial, or using pills to get back on course.

I often hear people confuse mind/body concepts, and thus misuse them. I had a conversation with a fellow physician wherein she stated that she could eat ice cream, and make it turn into broccoli with her mind. My point here is not that I doubt that the mind is powerful enough to do such a thing. As I stated in the previous chapter, "the spirit in which an act is conducted is more powerful than the act itself." However, there is a dilemma within this physician's outlook. She desires health, but in her reluctance to do those things that are consistent with health, she throws in a little rationalization. If she were, to be honest with herself, she could say, "This ice cream does not serve my body, it is not consistent with providing proper energy to my mind and body, but I am a good person for wanting to do what is appropriate for vitality." Pretending that ice cream, or cigarettes, for instance, is serving you, is going to create a dilemma. It demands rationalization, and rationalization is the precursor to stress. When you choose to eat candy, refrain from condemning yourself for your lack of willpower. Avoid justifying it with: "It's the only bad habit I still have." or "Anything in moderation is okay." Just say to yourself that you are aware that this food does not serve your body, but that you are a good person for being conscious of this.

Let's look at what Jesus thought about consumption. He said that it is not what you put in your mouth, it is what comes out of it that causes illness. If what comes out of your mouth is defensive or rationalizing, such as "I only eat ice cream once a month" or "It is the only thing that I do wrong," you are going to stay stuck.

Your dialogue is either working for you or against you (see the examples of Jesus, Gandhi, and Martin Luther King Jr. in section I). This is physics.

Just remember, an airplane is off course 90 percent of the time and remarkably gets to its destination. The pilots don't say "I can be off course and use my powerful mind to get us there," or "If I only turn left instead of right once in a while I will be fine..." Instead, they gently tell themselves that this is part of the process of getting to the destination, and they don't blame anyone or make excuses for themselves. The key is having the correct map (paradigm) and being willing to make corrections. Being optimistic or more importantly gentle while off course allows the correction.

Another dilemma that is so common today is that of money and happiness. The dilemma is the belief that the only way to be happy is to achieve a certain level in a career or attain material possessions. The dilemma with this is that making a lot of money most often takes a lot of time (i.e., overtime, a second job, mom working, etc.). In other words, something must give. The thing that usually gives way is something of value, such as family, or physical health. The rat race results in sacrificing the things that mean the most to you, with the expectation of being happy with all the money that you make. My patients assure me they value their children. But is a 60 or 70 or even 80-hour work week really valuing the children? Or is it valuing the money or power? Does it leave you time and energy to listen, talk, or play with your children?

When you ask people if they would rather be right or happy, most will answer "happy." The reality is quite different. I think everyone wants both... but won't admit it. Jesus said you can't serve two gods. He says you will love one and hate the other (Matthew 6:24).

Can you have money and simplicity? Can you have money and serve a higher power? Does money bring happiness? Does money create better health?

The answers to these questions have been answered in this book. We have to be open and abstract with answering them. It is not the money that brings happiness or health, it is the values and integrity that go along with attaining money that gives the pure happiness and health.

It is harder for a rich man to get through the eye of a needle than a poor man. This is not because to possess money or material things makes a man evil or anything of the sort. It is because of the false value the mind puts on these material things. It is difficult to have material things and not be attached to them. If you have difficulty in releasing them, then most likely you have made them your gods, and this will make healing impossible.

The irony of these teachings is that virtue and integrity in attaining wealth are paramount to achieving success in life.

When I ask my patients if they desire corrective care, they always say "Yes, of course." But inherent in correction, we always find the necessity for change.

Any dilemma can be eliminated by consistently practicing the exercises that follow. When you are willing to take responsibility, and by that, I mean to clarify your values, mission, and purpose, you will form the foundation for making the changes that serve you. Once you know why you are doing something, the "how" becomes easy.

SO WHERE DO ~~DOCTORS~~ TEACHERS FIT IN?

What has happened here is that doctors or treatments (external things) have, on a superficial level, made physical, visible changes in people's lives. Often they do work in masking the symptom, based upon the physiological reversal of secondary symptoms or secondary causes. If muscle tension is causing pain in your back, and massage, chiropractic or acupuncture relieves the pain temporarily (or even on a more permanent basis), it is accepted that the therapy or treatment produced increased blood flow, better nerve impulses, and lymphatic drainage resulting in the muscle relaxing. The science behind this reversal of symptoms is accepted yet fails many or most of the time in making the pain go away temporarily or more important permanently.

I can't count how many patients have this magical thinking when it comes to their symptoms. They are sedentary and/or overweight, or eating poorly, hate their jobs, have money problems. They get off the table from acupuncture or an adjustment and say, "It still hurts—you didn't get it all doc." I have looked inward with this and asked what am I doing that makes people think that I am a healer or have a magic wand? The thing that comes to mind is my ego getting stroked when people tell me how special I or my treatment is because of the time the headache or cramp that was with them for years went away with a pill I gave them. It could be easy for me to fall into the trap of being a hero but I don't want it for a minute. The biggest compliment I strive for is that a patient thanks me for guidance, support, knowledge, and connection.

When the doctor encourages the magical thinking that he has magic in his hands or special powers, people begin to think of the chiropractor as a miracle worker, or the drug as miraculous, or acupuncture as magic. This leads to people glorifying these entities in the same way they might revere their religion or money. The fact is that chiropractors and medical doctors know less about how to heal your body than the average person knows about quantum physics, astronomy, nuclear fusion, aeronautical engineering, horticultural and hairdressing put together. As Einstein said, "One thing I have learned in a long life, that all our science measured against reality, is primitive and childlike."

Most ailments or conditions require watchful waiting and a change in behavior and beliefs. Your true belief in healing (your lack of separation) can transcend the physical world and move to the next dimension; a headache would be gone or the back pain would stop. It is only your lack of belief that prevents this.

However, we are all at different stages of our spiritual journey. We must accept where we are in that journey. Attempting to take shortcuts could backfire. Use the nutritional therapy, chiropractic, or the medicine, and remind yourself that you have a healer within, and you did not inherit illness. You made it up, and you can dismiss it. Keep working on your questions. Ask why you made it up. When the time comes, your questions will have formed the basis for your forgiveness and subsequent healing. The key here is not to get caught up in believing that these philosophies are your new religion. I once heard an interesting saying that goes like this: Doctors will get off of their pedestals as soon as patients get off their knees.

The true meaning of doctor is a teacher. The meaning of physician is one who treats. As doctors, we must do what is in the best interest of our patients. We must empower them with knowledge, support, and guidance.

If you are willing to reshape your belief system as to where health really originates and apply timeless principles of nature in your day-to-day lifestyle, you can then look forward to little-to-no intervention from a physician.

This is the greatest gift a doctor (teacher) can give to you. It is the power to be certain that your health is within you, ready for you to access. All you need is faith. You might say, "But my faith is not strong enough." We were all born with enough faith to move mountains. You did not inherit illness. Your potential for health and healing is limitless. There is no doctor on this earth who can "fix" a patient. Think about cutting an apple in half, and suggesting to that same doctor that he make it whole again. Do you see the nonsense we are asking of our physicians? Perhaps you think your physician can reassemble an egg that has splattered to the ground. Where did we get the idea that a human being could accomplish these feats? Yet think how much, or how many, of your 60,000 thoughts a day are along those lines. I propose to you that when we are aligned with the truth, we are thinking with our purpose in mind. And the only way to think with purpose is to be willing.

Where the confusion starts is when, in the progression of a condition, the doctor aides the patient in temporarily reversing a stage of the condition by prescribing the right pill or giving the right treatment. A helpful analogy: your garden was not watered for several days and plants are starting to die. The doctor points this out to you and you add water. The plants respond... the doctor just educated and aided. The miracle is the plant's ability to recover.

STAGES OF ILLNESS

Even though the stages below follow the physiology and pathology taught in medical textbooks, healing often does not follow the same timelines. Relief care and temporary cures often follow the reverse of these stages:

Stage 1. Emotional (See The Course In Health Workbook)
- Vice over Virtue

Stage 2. Choice in Foods and or Stimulants
- Processed foods
- Fast food
- Overeating/over-drinking

- Over-working/stress

Stage 3. Accumulation
- Proteins. Putrefy
- Carbohydrates. Ferment
- Fats. Rancid

Stage 4. Intoxication
- Results of and Toxicity
- Body is trying to eliminate – Kidney, Lung, Colon, skin etc.
- Symptoms: Constipation, Diarrhea
- Stomach Problems
- Sinus Congestion
- Headache
- Colds, Immune Weakness
- Body Odor
- Skin Conditions (acne, etc.)

Stage 5. Deposition
- Accumulation of Toxins Overload
- Body's Defense Mechanism Can't Keep Up
- The Savings Account Is Being Over-drafted
- Pathology Begins: Abnormal Cell Function

Stage 6. Breakdown/Inflammation
- Hypertrophy and or Atrophy of Organ Function
- Toxic Matter Disturbing Organs and Joints
- Allergies, Autoimmune Conditions

Stage 7. Depletion of Energy Stores
- Adrenal Failure
- Blood Sugar Disturbances
- Internal Ulcers
- Virus / Fungus / Candida / Bacterial

Stage 8. Infiltrations or relocation
- Parasite, Fungal, Bacteria, Virus
- Illness, pain, change genetics

Stage 9. Decomposition then death

How treatment aides in reversing a stage, or blocking a symptom, can be explained. Important to understand is the difference between the reversal of the stage of illness and the blocking of a symptom. Drugs and surgery generally block symptoms. Herbs, food, exercise, and natural therapy sometimes reverse the stage of the disease. Also important to note is that healing does not require reversal of all symptoms. One key to this book and the workbook is to focus much if not all your attention on Stage 1 and the rest takes care of itself in most cases.

The creative intelligence who made the body is the force that is able to heal the body. Our faith, our ability to heal, has always been there, and shall always be there. Whether we access it is a different story. The healing that takes place when we cut ourselves is so miraculous that it cannot be reproduced by science. These are miracles that we are exposed to on a daily basis. Albert Einstein once said, ***"There are two ways to live your life. One is as though nothing is a miracle, the other is as though everything is a miracle."*** Marvel in the healing of a cut or the birth of a child and take these miracles and use them as a testimonial to your healing capacity as a child of wholeness. The only thing separating you from this is your own disbelief. Jesus never once *said* that he healed a person. People brought their children or themselves to his feet and they would be healed. What Jesus repeatedly said was "it is your faith that healed you." This probably confused people in those days as it does people today. Don't confuse His words, **your faith or your belief**. Without it, there is no healing; I call it your Grand Purpose. This is how we can explain spontaneous healing or spontaneous remissions.

Your doctor can help you heal if he encourages a patient's personal responsibility. Once again don't confuse healing with a cure. A cure is magic. Healing is a miracle. Everyone knows that magic is just an illusion; it is a smokescreen that is not real. It is temporary. Many doctors excel at these illusions by taking symptoms and covering them up with herbs, homeopathic remedies, drugs, adjustments, etc. These symptoms will always reappear in the same form or a different form if the patient continues to do or act in the same way that manifested the condition. As long as the true purpose of your illness has not been identified, healing will elude you. The true purpose of dis-ease is to teach, no more than this, but no less than this. If you embrace "internal" teachings you will embrace that illness is not real, and you will have access to the healing you truly desire. If your religion is your doctor, or drugs, or vitamins, then that is your god.

The storyline in the movie *Patch Adams* is how the mainstream medical system strives to create "gods" out of their doctors. It is **your** ego or separation that created this. It is **your** disbelief in **your** own power and therefore **your** need for someone else to do the work.

My investment in various university degrees in natural medicine and mainstream medicine are in excess of 8 years. At some point, I can't say exactly when I started asking questions. Questions like why are the best doctors in my field unable to get their patients well? Why does taking the right supplements, or poking a needle in the right place, not produce the health we are looking for? Taking an honest inventory of my life revealed to me that the only true way to help people is to not reinforce the incomplete way of thinking about health. Nothing I can do or prescribe is necessary for a patient's health.

In the true healing that I now seek, I am finally being honest with myself.

"Man cannot do well in one area of life whilst attempting to do wrong in another." Gandhi.

Encouraging people to take this or that supplement simply will not bring about the solution I know these people want.

If you perceive illness as the enemy, then it is. You make a condition real when you give it a name. You make a condition real when you defend it. You make a condition real when you fight it. As I said at the beginning of this book, a nation (or an individual) cannot simultaneously prepare for both war and peace. It is simple physics once again. Health insurance is really preparing for sickness. Thoughts about future illness (insurance) will produce illness, not health. Compare this to a nation which accumulates weapons for war "just in case." War WILL BE the product. Peace WILL NOT. Because the nation has not invested in peace, they have invested in war. So the atmosphere is now geared for war. Research on drugs simply creates more and more things to research about—it is self-perpetuating. Studies on herbs, looking for a "cure" no matter how benign, is simply busy work. Americans believe that technology rules. And to that extent it certainly does. But look what we have acquired because of our childish desires to find the shortcuts.

Did Jesus, Gandhi, the Dalai Lama or Buddha ever hint that the secret to healing could be discovered with technology or a pill? What all four leaders would have agreed on is that peace and healing are accessible to everyone on this planet at this very moment (no limiting time, circumstances, worthiness, or impossibility) whenever we as individuals choose to surrender to a higher power or the Grand Purpose.

THREE CHOICES

When asking patients what type of care they are looking for, I often ask what they would do if a little boy came into the room and started a small fire. Ninety-nine percent of the time the patient states they would put the fire out. I then ask what they would do if the same child came back five minutes later and started another. They usually say put the fire out then take the matches away from the child or find out why he is setting the fire. I then explain that your healthcare is similar. Relief care, which is drugs, vitamins, herbs, surgery, etc., is simply putting the fire out. Corrective care or healing is getting to the root of the problem by examining emotions, beliefs, and values, by way of prayer. To correct the problem with the child you would forget about the fire, for it will take care of itself and become smaller. Go directly to the child and discuss the issue and correct it.

You have three choices:

1. Chase fires in hopes that your fire department is always equipped (this will require a larger fire department as time goes on).
2. You can do both. Use external means to put the fire out, as you evaluate the external habit which caused the need for the fire.
3. You can correct the problem by changing your thoughts, beliefs, values, prayers, and meditation which will lead to mindful movement, mindful consumption, hygiene/sanitation, rewarding relationships, etc.

As long as patients believe that I myself, or the things I prescribe, are responsible for their health, they will balk at true healing. Without the shift in the responsibility we are still functioning within an incomplete paradigm.

Some say that most of the therapy currently being taught in schools actually *makes healing impossible.* The foundation of western law is based entirely upon the ancient code of Hammurabi, which is simply "an eye for an eye." I suggest to you that when a profession is based on revenge, it cannot lead you to spirituality. It cannot. **The end doesn't justify the means.** To repeat Gandhi's words, *"A man cannot do good in one area of his life whilst attempting to do wrong in another area. Life is one continuous whole."* It is interesting to note that Gandhi was a lawyer who gave up his profession for the truth. Gandhi had the knowledge to use violence for his means, but instead used non-violence. Albert Einstein said this about Gandhi: "Generations to come, it may be, will scarce believe that such a one as this ever in flesh and blood walked upon this earth." And Viscount Louis Mountbatten said, *"Mahatma Gandhi will go down in history on par with Buddha and Jesus Christ."* The reason I involve the law profession in this discussion is because it is so much a part of the western health system. Most doctors' actions are fear-based. Doctors fear the liability and many of their actions are based upon not getting sued. They are taught that they must take full responsibility for their patient's health. What is overlooked is the simple fact that the patient has need for a doctor because of their own choices; then, they want to blame that condition on luck, chance or genetics and therefore look for external remedies. The concept of suing a doctor for doing what you ask from them seems ridiculous. This is not to defend doctors. They are playing a role that is called for by the role the patients play. The scenario is a mutually satisfying, although completely useless, charade.

It is also interesting to note that the American population is experiencing the incredibly high amount of illness, obesity and chronic degenerative conditions. These illnesses are disproportionate to other cultures. The U.S. has the highest rates per capita of obesity, cancer, heart disease, arthritis, osteoporosis, depression, diabetes, and many other autoimmune and degenerative conditions. I present to you that one reason for this is because of the blaming habit we have cultivated.

When I was a kid, I would ask myself these questions when I wanted to decide on something important: 1) What would happen if everybody did this? 2) [the most important] Would I want someone else to do this to me? (a.k.a. the Golden Rule). If any of these do not sit well in your gut, the action you are contemplating probably doesn't assist you in your quest for wholeness.

CHANGING IS FOR YOUR GRAND PURPOSE

"Higher aims in themselves are more valuable, even if unfulfilled than lower ones quite attained." Goethe

This section has so much importance that it can't be stressed enough. I had so many committed and dedicated patients do fasts, change their lifestyle, start exercising—only to feel failure because their illness or condition remained. In my quest to find an answer, it became very clear that if the focus is external, the physics involved does not allow for healing. It becomes temporary and magic. I have been fortunate enough to be trained with a very select few of doctors on therapeutic fasting protocols. I, therefore, have been able to watch first-hand conditions and symptoms vanish during the fast: from psoriasis to hypertension and many other conditions. The primary factor of those whose symptoms did not return after a fast was in those patients who sought something beyond their physical condition. The belief in something greater than themselves. This is certainly not an easy endeavor but the need for a shift in consciousness is part of the process of success. It must start with the focus of the fast being an internal endeavor; NOT simply to remove an embarrassing skin condition or obesity. Rather, the actual goal is to become whole. This is like the person who endeavors to exercise/hike because he wants to experience nature which he values. The side effect is Whole Health versus the person forcing themselves to hike, run or walk to lose weight.

Whenever you endeavor to do an exercise program or diet, your underlying focus of the restraint or program is to serve your Grand Purpose.

Another example is that of participating in activities: eating, exercise, work, etc. (i.e. If you exercise with an internal framework – you love it, time flies by, nobody will stop you in the exercise, you make time for it). The person who exercises because their belly is too big is coming from an external framework and will not see results.

For the rest of us, we must examine why we do a fast or a vegan diet or exercise which results in lowering blood pressure, reversing inflammation, etc. We must step back and ask: are we doing it to reduce pain (external) or heal (internal)? If it is to heal we must consider the cause… which is always a separation from our higher power, and sin that leads to the manifestation of the condition. If the cause is wrong thinking or separation then the healing is unity and love. The exercise or the diet is commonsense tools to get you back to unity only if achieved in an intrinsic way.

The question is why do some heal without doing the exercise program or the diet? This crucial question helps to uncover the purpose of "doing" things like diet and exercise to heal. Proactive steps like diet and exercise must be distinguished from "magic" like things that cover up symptoms. Many natural and most mainstream medical treatments cover up symptoms and create more separation and make healing impossible. The difficulty is determining between symptom care (magic care) and steps to healing. In brief, symptom care is external. Healing is internal. Fasting, diet, exercise, etc. are not treatments and are in no way covering symptoms. The focus on which an act is conducted is more powerful than the act itself.

Please don't confuse the fact that these internal actions are not the cause of the condition… the cause being separation, sin or wrong thinking that led you to conditions of the body. Going full circle it is why not all people need to diet or exercise to heal. Remember that healing is permanent and cure is temporary. Healing is a miracle that unites; the cure is magic that separates.

It is difficult to imagine or believe that it is NOT the diet or exercise that heals a person. For most the deductive reasoning and connection between doing a diet, taking herbs, or exercising and the abatement of symptoms or a condition seems hard to refute. The fact is that if this were the case all conditions would be healed with diet and exercise. The focus in which an act is conducted is more powerful than the act itself. This means that the person doing a vegan diet without the values and intention to heal on a spiritual level by changing from vice to virtue will never heal.

Jesus said, "It is easier for a camel to go through the eye of a needle than for someone who is rich to enter the kingdom of God" (Matthew 19:24). The reason being if your money is your god, or food, or exercise, or treatments, or pills you will not access you Grand Purpose. To put this in real life meaning, my interpretation is that money is not evil if you serve your true purpose, however it is difficult to have both because serving one creates a need to focus on that ONE. If you take emotion out of it, you can see some that do not make their surgery, their doctor or pills their god and can access their Grand Purpose. The dilemma is that if you choose to fix the problem with pills, surgery, etc. you will be disregarding your own power to heal. Ask yourself if you know people who love to exercise and use it to serve their Grand Purpose versus those who use exercise as a religion (same question with diet and food). When you serve a Grand Purpose, you respect the food, give gratitude, eat pure and clean and do it for your Grand Purpose—not to reduce your weight or get rid of a condition.

The short-term gains while doing special diets of water-only fasts are irrefutable. I have personally seen hypertension drop 90 points over the fast. I have witnessed psoriasis that covers someone's arms, and legs go completely away with a fast. There are many other examples. The intrinsic part of allowing the body to heal is amazing. Why then does the high blood pressure sometimes return or the skin problems erupt? It's not luck or chance. If internal change did not happen on an emotional level, if the addiction was not addressed, I propose it was "magic."

TESTIMONIALS AKIN TO THE MULTILEVEL SCHEME

There is a destructive aspect inherent in the way testimonials are used in business through marketing and advertising. The purpose is to sell something. The underlying message is that this product or service will make you happy or healthy or both – with very little to no effort. Whenever I hear testimonials of this sort, I cringe. It is how most multi-level companies or pharmaceutical companies abuse the external to sell. Even if it is well-intentioned, it is misleading and destructive. On the contrary, a testimonial that has its basis in hard work, change, and action is constructive, but there seems to be a very small market for these items.

I believe the testimonial is built on a house of cards. It takes the 1 or 2 percent of people who lose weight (or who benefit by coincidence, placebo, or maybe the product), and then build on low percentage as if it were 100 percent. The problem is it has no foundation. The purpose of the testimonial is to overcome the fact that the product or service needs artificial support and focus unethically on those very small cases of success. Luckily the FTC (Federal Trade Commission) is regulating these deceptive advertising techniques more and more. The main reason I am so dead set against testimonials is that they are the epitome of using external means.

Looking for a quick fix is a waste of your time. It is a vice. Once you realize this, you will be ready to change. When I recommend my patient's supplements, adjustments and other quick fixes that come across as external if the true cause is not addressed. These things only lead patients to believe that there is hope for external treatments. I hope is to show people that doing the work will result in solid answers that are lasting. The goal is to look at the fire and go directly to the cause. Ignoring the fire is hard for many to do because of their beliefs. The difference between treatments being external versus internal is how they are delivered. If the doctor is the all-knowing guru or the supplement or drug is mystical, it is external. If the patient comes in with the attitude "fix me" … again, it is external. When intrinsic treatments are explored, we can facilitate healing.

Consider the following analogy to help describe the insanity of quick fixes. Make believe that all doctors (natural and medical) were held to the same standards and ethics of bridge building engineers. If an engineer knew that some action in the building of a bridge was defective, he would change it right away. If he knew about defects already in existence he would start from the beginning and would not compromise. There is no such thing as a band-aid for this field. Imagine doctors acting in the same professional way that engineers do: every doctor would tell their patient that giving them this drug/vitamin/surgery is unethical and then he is doing them a disservice. As a doctor, I know that the cause is from your day-to-day choices. Just like the engineer, if I help you cover it up, I am an accomplice?

First, do no harm. In any ethical medical research, if there appears to be any harm to the subjects, the research must be stopped immediately. This applies to all research, pharmaceuticals, natural supplements, surgery, etc. Are doctors doing harm upon patients if the harm is not as immediate yet more insidious?

To treat or not to treat? A shocking 80 percent of problems require no treatment needed for both mainstream medical and natural care.

The unintended evil of marketing and advertising is at a peak. From the vantage of a new business wanting to spread the word of their presence, you would think advertising and marketing are essential and benign. Informative advertising without tactic geared sales is necessary - like having a sign in front of a business, passing out menus, or listing your services or bios of employees.

However, the reality is that 99 percent of advertising and marketing is geared towards the external: external and separation. It is fear, guilt and worthiness triggered. It isn't intended to inform the consumer; it is to sell at any cost. Think about things that have intrinsic value; very seldom are they advertised or have marketing campaigns. Why do we not see ads or marketing for the Bible or the Koran? Why do the best doctors, dentists, hairdressers, etc., not advertise? Why are the shadiest of medications and medical procedures in advertisements such as magazines and television? Why are legal drugs the second most item advertised? (second to automobiles).

The honest answer is that the advertiser and marketer have the drug dealer mentality: "If I don't do it someone else will." There is also very little consideration for whether the product or service is needed for the person being targeted.

The expert in marketing hired by the drug or vaccine company is NOT a doctor versed in microbiology and immunology. Their degree is in selling the product without the discernment of need. How they sell is the psychological tactics used to brainwash people. Hey! It works and puts food on their table, right? But it doesn't address the deeper issue of your health and healing? The purpose of addressing this is so you the customer of healthcare can step back and ask if you are the target of sales that elicit your external weak spots. For example, a weak spot may be fear - or another weak spot may be to blame, this condition is not my fault and this drug is magic, it's safe because this doctor (actor) is telling me so, if it's on TV it must be safe and true.

SECTION 10

ACCEPT AND EMBRACE YOUR CONDITION

Trusting in the Process - The Focus is the Outcome

If we perceive illness as the enemy, then it is. It is all in our perception. If we only see health, energy, and vitality, then that is all there is. You make a condition real when you give it a name. You make a condition real when you fight it. You make a condition real when you defend it. The Workbook offers lessons on how your emotions, thoughts, and feelings give you the insight to your Focus.

Two causes of illness: 1) Thinking about a condition. 2) Negative emotions which lead us to unhealthy choices. Unhealthy choices and negative emotions cause illness. Remember illness is purposeful and meaningful. There is a lesson to learn from it.

People try to avoid the pain. They may use drugs, surgery, herbs, acupuncture, or the latest fad. All it does is delay the healing. Remember: cures are magic and temporary. Healing is the miracle and is forever. Our goal should not be healthy; it should be what health provides us in achieving immortality - through love.

Relationships are the tool we have to work on in our spirituality. There is no growth or healing without a relationship. All healthy, fulfilling relationships have one common denominator: intrinsic qualities of respect, honesty, laughter, and trust (in contrast to the relationship built for the short term based upon looks, body or money).

When you are ready to heal, you will bring special people into your life. These people are your spiritual companions. Understanding the importance of and valuing special relationships serves your health and happiness. To heal is to unite with those like you.

Your relationships speed up your journey to healing if you appreciate them as purposeful. The irony is that the struggles we have in relationships with our parents/spouses/ neighbors/co-workers that bring out illness ultimately serve the purpose of strengthening the relationships with ourselves if only we look inside.

When embracing your condition, first observe the beliefs that were in place when you created it. Examine them and understand they were your companion on the path to the illness. You must identify the beliefs before you can release them. Forgive yourself for inviting them along, before your healing can begin.

Our human experience is but a total of our past experiences. These experiences have shaped our lives, without a doubt. We are now ready to take those experiences and form different beliefs from them, which will allow us to enter this complete paradigm of health and apply it to a broader definition of health. This new definition will include healthy relationships, career, spiritual, social, mental, physical, etc. By using these same principles of the complete paradigm of health (that is, an internal manifestation of internal healing) we are escaping a belief system which must by its very nature foster dilemmas. When you apply these principles to all areas of your life, you will put yourself in tune with healing. I believe we have the keys—in our pockets—where they do no good. Take them out and try them on the various doors in your life. The correct door is the complete paradigm of life which will produce health. Entering the door requires virtues.

It is here where we make a clear distinction between a cure and true healing. A cure is something that is temporary or magic. It is unreal, much like our physical body. And like our physical body, it can't defy time. Healing is of the mind and transcends the physical (time) and is lasting. Healing takes place when we surrender the ego, and stay in the process of unconditional love. Healing takes place by way of praying spontaneously to our Creator, with gratitude for that which we already have. The key to forgiveness is forgiveness directed to our own being. We are taught external forgiveness or ego forgiveness; I suggest internal forgiveness. The concept of forgiveness of others, I believe, is a human misinterpretation. To forgive others is simply an external compromise, which further separates and fuels the ego. It is both impossible and unnecessary to forgive anyone other than you.

Prayer and forgiveness are essential for freedom and healing, unity, and deeper consciousness.

Forgiving outside of yourself will tempt you to look externally for fault thus making exceptions. I often hear: *But what about a baby that gets in a car accident?* She didn't ask for it: It is external, etc. Or what about having to forgive a rapist? And so on. When you let go of the instinct to forgive outside of yourself, all the gray areas will melt away. Do not use hypothetical or outside examples to prove to yourself that your case is external and not your fault.

So often people feel bad about their condition: embarrassed that they have a mental condition, breast cancer, or heart disease. This embarrassment is merely guilt. First look inside to find out where this is coming from. For example, consider a person who has just recently found they have heart disease, in the past, this person may have judged others who have had heart disease as being angry or fat or simply not taking care of their health. When they are put in this same group that they have prejudged they may feel embarrassed, therefore they might rationalize with external excuses. All these feelings will not allow for healing and change.

The bald eagle is unique in the way it reacts to the challenge of a storm. Ordinary birds will do one of two things: Either they will stay and try and fight the storm or take shelter and hide. This is what most people do when faced with a problem, which we will call a storm. The bald eagle has a twist. He rises above the storm. The people who rise above their storm will see a spontaneous remission, manifesting as health, happiness, and healing.

When we study the universe and physics, it is undeniable that the universe is one whole. Therefore, we cannot separate our universe from our creator and say that our creator is not in everything. So if our creator is in everything, and we are connected to the universe then you essentially have all the power. Attacking your body with drugs (pharmaceutical or recreational), vitamins, or other treatments is separating yourself from that oneness. It is essentially saying you are smarter than your creator. When separation is ended, true healing will occur.

Nearly every person who enters a doctor's office wants reassurance that they are okay, and that their condition is not their fault. They want the doctor to empathize with them that they are doing their part to deserve perfect health, and all they need to do is take this pill or follow through with this treatment. They want to be told that they don't have to change their lives and it's not their fault. They invest great amounts of time and money in finding the doctor who will say this in the most convincing manner. One major issue taught at practice management seminars is to make the patient feel good when they leave. They are in the office because they hurt. They are coming to you to make it go away. However, the doctor can't because the doctor didn't create the dis-ease. The question I will ask my patients frequently is whether they think that they can be healthy without being happy. They will answer "NO". The indisputable logic within this framework is this: it is not possible to fix a condition by addressing physiology alone. One must address the mental/emotional or spiritual being as well. Disease starts in the mind and eventually manifests in physical form. Therefore, anything the body produces or does not produce is secondary to the true cause. For example, the reason you have breast cancer is not truly because of pesticides in your food or the amount of animal fat you have eaten throughout your life. The reason you have breast cancer is because you chose to engage in certain behaviors in the first place. You may say, "But I didn't know that these things were not good for me! Why didn't my doctor tell me?! And if that is so, then why don't my friends have breast cancer?" You are on your own journey. Your body is telling you what you need to learn. Your body is not the messenger for your friends. Their own bodies are speaking to them.

If your doctor puts you outside of your comfort zone, if he has made you think, or if he has placed the responsibility of your health and happiness in your hands, he has done you a service.

TIME & SPACE

Next to death, Time is probably one of the most perplexing concepts. The concept of time is connected to the concept of space. Time is measured by motion and can be circular or linear. I propose time for the purpose of health to be circular. Like cause and effect being thought of as linear, I propose that cause and effect is also circular with cause determining effect while effect creating cause by its effect.

We look to *save* time doing some things and *value* time in others. We want time to pass when doing things we perceive as uncomfortable or don't enjoy. We experience time as "standing still" or "flying by" when we are in flow. Flow meaning doing things we love and are passionate about—consistent with being on purpose. This makes time not exist. Watching your favorite show, or engaging in an activity you love. Flow is truly internal and connected to your Grand Purpose.

When it comes to separation, sin, addiction or the vice… we can simplify by saying we are "wasting time." Otherwise said: we miss the mark. The Grand Purpose simply saves time.

"Time seems to go forward, but it is really going backward to the point at which time began." A Course in Miracles (ACIM)

Time and space have no meaning in infinity.

DEATH & BIRTH

As an end or beginning, death is inevitably a part of our life. Birth has a lot of the same properties as death. We come into this world and gasp for air; and at this moment we form a sort of independence and connection with the world and universe: by breathing the air particles and consuming the finite water particles within our universe. Many have suggested we should make the birthing experience for our children a natural process. Many women strive to labor and deliver naturally without drugs, to allow their child to enter this world peacefully and better connect with their mother. Some question why a mother would choose to embrace the pain of labor and delivery versus having drugs to block the pain. I insist these women (NONE of them) are not trying to be martyrs or anything of the sort. They simply want the best for their child and also the best for themselves. Having a vaginal, drug-free birth is proven to produce a healthier child. This helps mother and child. Besides this, there is also a spiritual benefit that is gained in allowing and embracing the "pain" of labor. The process of birthing is a complicated process of simply letting go and connecting with oneness.

This same process of letting go is seen in the process of dying. It is a process, labor, and a journey.

If you live life with a higher purpose, are open to change, and grow more virtuous with meaningful relationships and love… embrace death like natural birth and let go. Otherwise, there is as much to fear in death as there is in birth (See step 3 in The Course In Health Workbook).

"Everything living strives for wholeness" Carl G. Jung

If we look at the meanings behind Easter and Death and connect it with sin and illness, and cause and effect—we come to the conclusion that disease is not real—nor is the sin.

SIN & THROWING STONES
"Hate the sin, not the sinner" Mahatma Gandhi

Sin is not guilt. Sin is not evil. It is simply going against our virtues. We can sin by choosing the vice over the virtue and each time it will give us feedback. Sin is a thought or action directed towards the vice. The Greek translation is "to miss the mark." We can use the outcome (feelings/results/effect) of sin as the failure that leads us to success. That feedback is purposeful and meaningful. Sin wastes time, it causes pain, AND guides us back to health.

"That we call sin on others we call experiment for us." Ralph Waldo Emerson

In Cause and Effect, sin causes sickness and death. In the workbook, we get to the root "cause." The ultimate connection between sin and death—and time and space—are the lessons taught by Buddha, Jesus, and Mohammed.

"All things appear and disappear because of the concurrence of causes and conditions. Nothing ever exists entirely alone; everything is in relation to everything else." Buddha

THOUGHTS ARE THINGS

"Nothing real can be threatened. Nothing unreal exists. Herein lies the peace of God." A Course in Miracles

The fact is that our thoughts are material things. In physics, thoughts can be identified as subtle vibrations of energy—making thoughts real "things." This became real to me after taking college level physics courses. Because we do not see radio waves that deliver music or news doesn't mean that radio waves are not real things. When something is tangible it becomes more real in our minds. We can then take beliefs, feelings, thoughts, and words and start looking at them as tangible, real and changeable. Words are translated to thoughts, both conscious and subconscious. It is crucial that we choose healing words (See The Course In Health Workbook step 1).

"There was never anything that did not proceed from a thought."
Ralph Waldo Emerson

PROFOUND SIMPLICITY

Consider stopping the intellectualizing of health and just experience it. This complete paradigm is a simple one. We all have health and happiness. Simplicity is not getting caught up in the technological way. Simplicity may be a great challenge if you don't have purpose and values. When people look for their health and happiness outside of themselves they are moving away from simplicity. The opposite of simplicity is complexity.

"A calm and modest life brings more happiness than the pursuit of success combined with constant restlessness." Albert Einstein

THE BEGINNING

We must start with the end in focus, which becomes the beginning. *We are born into a world of nature, our second birth is into the world of spirit.* Bhagavad-Gita

What you have experienced, no power on earth can take from you. - Victor Frankl.

The purpose of this book is to join with those who are looking for a better way—the people who are willing to take responsibility for their lives.

Jesus said it is harder for a rich man to get through the eye of a needle, than to get into heaven. I say it is harder for someone utilizing external means to get through an eye of a needle, than to experience true healing.

In 1948 General Omar N. Bradley said, *"We have too many men of science, too few men of God. We have grasped the mystery of the atom and rejected the Sermon on the Mount."* He continued by saying *"Ours is a world of nuclear giants and ethical infants. We know more about war than we know about peace, more about killing than we know about living."* The irony is that our healthcare is not scientific.

To quote a man who is undoubtedly the most scientifically advanced man to live on this earth, Albert Einstein said, *"a country cannot simultaneously prepare for war and peace at the same time."* He also said *"One thing I have learned in a long life, that all our science measured against reality, is primitive and childlike."* The obvious step is you can't prepare for illness and health at the same time.

"May your Aim be the good of All." Bhagavad Gita

PRAYER & FORGIVENESS

We must look at the true cause (not the secondary cause, the proximate cause or symptom). Prayer and forgiveness address the true cause. For me, this goes back to grade nine religion class with my teacher Mr. White whom I respected very much. He taught us something about forgiveness that has stuck with me. It was that forgiveness is about forgiving yourself, and that true forgiveness forgets. When this happens, we stop being the victim and we connect with our deeper self. We become gentle towards our separation that has caused the illness and reconnect. I believe that when you connect at this level you emanate love and you heal.

The greatest gift we have available to us is prayer. Prayer is the single most effective method we have of changing. Prayer is giving thanks, the process of forgiveness, and living in the process. Prayer asks for nothing. It is communication without attachment to outcome. It is sublimation to the divine power within ourselves, which is inherent within all of us. Prayer asks simply for the ability to receive what is already ours, to accept what is already there. We no longer remind God to give us what we think we need. Instead, we remind ourselves to hear with the ears we have, touch with our hands, smell with our nose, see with our eyes, love with our heart. It asks that we be awakened to what is real. It provides us with the ability to unite. It teaches us to forgive ourselves for our separateness. It helps us live in the process.

So what is healing? Healing is the process of surrendering the ego. It is overcoming separation. It is taking responsibility. To heal is to unite with people and things that are like you. It is praying. It is forgiving. Prayer and forgiveness are both the process and the outcome of healing. I believe the insight in this book along with surrounding yourself with people who engender joy in your life, can help you achieve the state of being happy and healthy... being whole.

I know there are other roads to happiness and health. Since time began, it has been man's ultimate quest. "Hitting the wall" or "bottoming out" physically was most often the catalyst for people to change and heal. In this process, we become whole and virtuous.

- Forgive
- Love
- Give Thanks
- Let Go

"God Grant Me The Serenity To Accept The Things I Cannot Change, Courage To Change The Things I Can, And Wisdom To Know The Difference." - Niebuhr

Going back to time being either linear or circular: If prayer is circular and not linear, it is better understood that it asks for nothing.... The sick believe healing is the enemy. What the sick believe will help will hurt them, what they believe will harm will help. They mourn their sickness and rejoice in it. The sick are a part of the movie instead of watching the movie. The sick believe in guilt and punishment—prayer transcends this.

ATTRIBUTES OF THE WHOLE

The 80 percent of the population who have money problems, the 80 percent of the population who have relationship problems, the 80 percent of the population who have health problems, have issues with virtues and addictions.

You *can* stop blaming and choose *virtues* to join the 20 percent who are healed or healing in these areas. The path to virtues is a gentle one. We can blame our teachers, parents, and doctors for creating sickness—or we can change our belief and use the new map of health to break free. If you want to change your life, *YOU* need to change your life.

Those looking on and wishing they had millions of dollars or had great health or the perfect spouse are missing the ONE thing. Each of these requires the virtues to live accordingly. The virtues that the ill refuse to admit, change and grow into. What this book is not, is a dream or promise of a quick fix. It is a guide to health, wealth and happiness, through virtues.

MONEY
- Their close friends have financial control and success.
- They have a mentor.
- They read daily
- They set goals and track them.
- They watch little TV.

- They watch their words & thoughts.
- They don't set limits. They think big.
- They don't give up.
- They are positive.
- They educate themselves.
- They attribute their success to internal attributes.

RELATIONSHIPS
- Their close friends have solid relationships and share similar values.
- They see their relationships in a positive light.
- They commit time and energy to their relationships.
- They affirm - versus - invalidate.
- They don't blame. They fight fair.
- They allow their relationships to express their feelings – Good communication.
- They are optimistic towards their partner.
- They have their own interests and take care of themselves.
- They trust and respect.
- Most important they love themselves.

HEALTH
- Their close friends have health.
- They don't eat a lot.
- They eat whole foods – They don't diet.
- They are active.
- They don't sweat the small stuff.
- They work in a job they love.
- They work on themselves.
- They believe health comes from within.

The healthy move towards pleasure and do so from an internal focus. The sick move away from pain and blame with an external focus.

To heal is to unite and connect with those like you. Thank each relationship, experience, pain, and illness as a part of the Grandness of your experiences. May the workbook that follows gently guide you to what is already present.

The words "health," "whole," and "holy," are all derived from the Anglo-Saxon word root: "Hal." "Healing" is derived from the same word root and means... to restore to a state of wholeness, soundness, or integrity.

The workbook that follows is the difference maker. It's the place where this book and other self-help or health books are polar opposites. Most self-help books do not require the "mess" required to make the change and become whole; similar to those that want a nice dinner and don't want to make a mess in the kitchen. We all know that the mess is required to make that special dinner. The same mess is required to get to health. It is in the eye of the beholder whether the mess is painful or the pain is overlooked by the joy of the outcome. For myself, the mess in the kitchen is a path to a great meal. This is the same feeling I have in dealing with my (mess) stuff, leading to health and happiness. The biggest attribute or common denominator of this section is the willingness to do the work.

THE SWAMP VERSUS THE TEMPLE
"Have no friend not equal to yourself" **Confucius**

The question of the swamp attracting the mosquito is a simple one. The swamp attracts mosquitoes, virus, victims, addicts and the like. Does the swamp reflect you or do you reflect the swamp?

The claim of the germ theory being flawed is based upon sound science: immunology and microbiology and clinical science. The microbiologist that refuses to look at the host is as ridiculous as a congressman or president focusing on bullets as the cause of gun deaths. The bullet is akin to the virus. It is one of the last things implicated and very shortsighted to believe in a bullet theory or germ theory.

It is well accepted that a virus mutates a gene which in turn may cause a thing some call cancer. If we don't start with the swamp in this obvious deductive reasoning we focus on the shortsighted virus, genes, and bullets as the cause of death theory. The amount of money wasted on fighting cancer-based upon this flawed theory and short-sighted thinking is not wasted; it can be used to show the insanity. I don't get upset at these failures, I just use them to point out how the amount of wasted spending has resulted in failure. This failure leads us to a more complete focus on cancer or victim. All those dollars spent on cancer research and genes help prove how flawed the germ theory is. Thank you to all the well-intentioned researchers and geneticists clearly showing that the answer is much deeper in the cause.

The same focus on addictions and mental conditions apply. The virus is the alcohol and the host blaming or being victim to the alcohol (virus). The alcohol is of little significance to a healthy, whole person. Many people pass bars and liquor stores each day to return home to healthy relationships or go to the temple instead.

Next, we apply the same to wasted counseling services which label the virus (mental condition) and pity the swamp. A little confusing for some but the analogy holds true. Remember that the swamp has a purpose. The swamp creates fresh water and oxygen, help clean water etc.

The perpetrator attracts the victim; otherwise said: the swamp attracts the mosquito. We can all agree that the perpetrator selects the victim by subtle nonverbal cues from posture, gait, or an overall energy.

For any person claiming that I am blaming the victim please stop it. It is a misrepresentation and a manipulation of what I am saying. Do I blame the influenza virus or the bullet? Absolutely not. They are, however, obviously linked to the cause. If the swamp is the mosquito and vice versa, and the perpetrator is the victim, we can see it's a cycle. It is accepted that these bugs are opportunistic and important in the cycle of life.

Perhaps we can agree that all perpetrators were at one time a victim. You don't become violent without exposure to mistrust and abuse. The perpetrator's way of dealing with past abuse is to abuse others before they get hurt. Another fact is that some people exposed to mistrust and abuse may allow others to abuse them and tolerate it, while others who have been abused will retreat and avoid intimacy or relationships out of fear. Healthy people do not attract abusive people; they do not tolerate abuse or put off the energy that they are the target or a victim. For those stuck on blame, I will entertain... Let's go back to the hot tub analogy or the rundown person (host) being a suitable environment for a virus. We all agree that a hot tub ignored for 6 months turns into a swamp and attracts the virus (mosquito). We also agree that the rundown person is a suitable environment for the virus (Influenza A). Are you still calling this blame? Change it to a purpose and we all heal. The purpose of attracting the influenza virus is purposeful—to restore the person back to homeostasis and balance—by creating a fever and slowing the person down, making them hydrate and change. Would you still call this blame? Heck no! So when the perpetrator attracts the victim, it is purposeful and intended to create wholeness. When the victim attracts the perpetrator, same applies.

The same can be said about "negative" emotions: Worry, fear, anger, etc. are purposeful "swamp" emotions that if addressed in a healthy, gentle, honest way, will lead to healing.

PHYSICIAN HEAL THYSELF

I got into medicine, I thought, to help people. After the sincere work I have done in my career—alongside the relationships, I have formed, the counsel I have given, and alongside of the joys and pains I have felt—the one thing that stands out the most is that you can't love someone if you don't love yourself. Healing is a descriptive act, the same as loving; it can only be done with internal focus. No person can heal another. They can only heal themselves. I have been humbled by shifting from an external perspective to connecting to my internal guidance in my own process of growth. I owe this to all of my relationships, my **Grand Purpose** and the *Beatitudes.*

THE EMOTION-LINK

Life traps include illness. The following questionnaire reveals your personal traps. The

Secondary Gains: General

- Subconscious need for dependence: "I will get cared for or get attention." ... "My turn."
- Subconscious need for dependence with revengeful feelings: "I will get paid my salary and don't have to work" ... "I was so unappreciated" ... "They owe me."
- Subconscious need to maintain or exert family status, entitlement, control, appreciation, etc. (i.e. feel controlled, getting ill allows for control)
- A desire for preferential treatment at work, home, and/or sympathy and reason to not have to work.
- Subconscious or conscious desire for sympathy and attention from family and friends.
- A way to back out of unpleasant, uncomfortable, painful life roles. (Caring for kids, parents, yard work, etc.)
- Ability to become the center of attention without asking for it.
- Subconscious way to salvage a relationship. "He will not leave me now."
- Subconscious way to reignite love, excitement in the family.
- A way to dominate or control family and friends. A way to stop family fighting, tension or conflict.
- Something to talk about. "My condition is special, grandiose, the worst." When bored illness gives you something to do and talk about. (Dr. visit, and dinner conversation)
- Approval and validation from the doctor. Touch and listening from the doctor. My husband does not listen to me, my naturopath or MD listens.
- Receive legal drugs with no guilt or shame.

My secondary gains from my illness, physical condition and or life traps.:
*hard to impossible for you to consciously be aware of the secondary gain and or emotional link. The following pages (your traps and or condition) give you the insight to likely secondary gains linked to your trap or condition.
* read the Secondary gain and temporary admission in the lists below that relate to you. Then wait a couple of minutes and without reviewing write down what you remember. Otherwise said...List your emotional-link to your condition.

ABANDONED - UNWANTED

Secondary Gain: I don't have to commit myself. I won't get hurt if I don't commit. I can blame the person leaving for my non-committal. See, they left me.

Temporary Admission: I am non-committal (not my partner), I am unwanted, I am abandoning, I am unconnected, closing off.

Goal: I am committed and wanted. It is safe to love and be loved. When I commit it will mirror back to me.

Purpose: Constructive aspect to feeling abandoned is to get commitment needs met or become committed. While at the same time protecting yourself. The destructive aspect is being not committing and being unavailable.

Vice to Virtue: Peace, Connected, Unwavering, Committed, Open.

ADRENAL

Secondary Gain: Time to rest. I have an excuse for failure because I am exhausted. Being defeated is painful so I need a reason to rest.

Temporary Admission: I am exhausted(ing), I am defeated(ing), I am competing, I blame myself, I am hard on myself, I am going in the wrong direction, off track.

Goal: I don't need to compare myself to others to win. I have self-control. I am at ease.

Purpose: Balanced hormones for stress, survival, and sexuality. When I control blood sugar, burn protein and fat, I can react to stressors like illness or injury.

Vice to Virtue: Courage, Strength, Diligence, Humility.

ALCOHOLISM or ABUSE

Secondary Gain: Numb painful feelings. Give you confidence, temporary high, stress relief, and escape responsibilities. Subconsciously punish yourself. (**see above)

Temporary Admission: I am running away, I want to escape, I am unable to cope, I feel shame, guilt, and or self-rejection. I do not love myself, what is the use. I am dependent on others. I feel anxious and unstable. I am impulsive.

Goal: I am open to resolving negative emotions, I feel worthy, I have a purpose, I confront my fears. I am at peace.

Purpose: Alcohol craving and consumption are directly related to hypoglycemia and stress. With increased stress, our bodies require increased sugar(alcohol). Alcohol requires no digestion and is absorbed easily. The purpose of consuming is to satisfy hypoglycemia and provide a dopamine response and high. It is a part of the fight and flight response. It's necessary to cope with stress.

Alcohol abuse and addiction serves to feed the hypoglycemia and stress and give you a high to avoid the pains and emotions you run from.

Vice to Virtue: Courage, Strong, Confident, Diligence, Connected

See Undisciplined.

ALLERGIES

Secondary Gain: Protection from the irritant, excuse to stay away from the irritant.

Temporary Admission: It is not safe to express my feelings, it is easier to blame the substance then confront the fear.

Goal: I am confronting my fears, I accept my power.

Purpose: An immune response to a stimulus you have an issue with. Being allergic to the substance relieves me from my fears temporarily.

Vice to Virtue: Temperance, Peace, Fair, Connected.

See Depression & Anxiety.

ANKLES: FEET/TOES
Secondary Gain: If I don't have to make decisions I will be safe.
Temporary Admission: I am inflexible, I am not stable, I worry about the direction and the future, I feel anxious.
Goal: I am flexible and stable, I let go of my need to control the details of the future.
Purpose: To give stability and details to the direction we are going. To move through life with ease. Give balance.
Vice To Virtue: Strong, Balanced, Diligence.
Toes: Details And Direction.
Big Toe: Stability.
Second: Fear.
Middle: Sex and Anger.
Fourth: Grief.
Little: Family.
Ankles: Right: Money And Details **Left:** Relationship And Details.
Feet: Self-awareness, Sensations, and Feelings.

ANXIETY
Secondary Gain: If I have control I am safe. I use worry to justify my control issues. If I worry bad things don't happen. (**see above)
Temporary Admission: I want to be in control to feel safe, I don't trust. I am dependent, I am untrusting. I am compulsive; If I don't do it myself, people will let me down. People are out to get me.
Goal: I let go of my need for control, I trust in the process, I trust myself and the people around me.
Purpose: To tell you there is a threat, real or perceived. Anxiety indicates danger. We must differentiate from personal and impersonal. If Anxiety is not addressed, the destructive aspect is cognitive distortions or judgments creating problems in your life.
Vice to Virtue: Balance, Diligence, Connected, Peace, Strong.

ARTHRITIS
Secondary Gain: I can be stiff and rigid in my movement and thinking. I can be right by criticizing and judging others. I feel good to be right, but need to continue to feed the source. I am able to feel inflamed. (Feeling) Being right feels good.
Temporary Admission: I am rigid, I am critical, I am inflexible. I need to be right. I am angry, +hostile.
Goal: To be flexible, I am gentle, I am peace, I want to be happy.
Purpose: arthritis is related to inflammation. Think of inflammation as fire. It is a response to irritants, damaged cells, and or pathogens. The inflammatory response is a defensive action to protect you, not harm you. In summary, the protection is by making a joint stiff and painful to not use while you address what is *inflaming* the joint. Alcohol, cigarettes, sugar are like gasoline on the fire and further cause the inflammation. However, when you get to the Emotion-Link and address that link it is the beginning of anti-inflammation. Where the inflammation targets are no mistake.
Right side: Of the body Masculine.
Left Side: Of the body Feminine. When breakdown or inflammation predominates on one side look too masculine-feminine imbalance.
See Emotion-link for hands, versus ankles, neck, versus spine, etc. The destructive aspect is obviously crippling.
Vice to Virtue: Forgiveness, Gratitude, Open, Peace, Purity, Patience, Temperance

AUTOIMMUNE

Secondary Gain: Working against yourself: body attacks its own tissue. Attacking myself prove s that I am not loveable. It's not my fault. (**see above)

Temporary Admission: Holding on to childhood trauma. I am working against myself, I am attacking myself, I reject who I am.

Goal: Be gentle on myself, I love myself, I am accepting myself.

Purpose: the immune system is to create immune responses against dangers. When the body thinks of itself as a danger it wants to destroy or reject itself.

Vice to Virtue: Forgiving, Diligence, Patience, Connected, Competent.

Rheumatoid arthritis: Bitter and rigid.

Lupus: What is the use (thyroid).

Inflammatory bowel disease: Obsessive.

Multiple sclerosis: Control, stuck, poor me.

Psoriasis: Not responsible, blame, hate.

Hashimoto's Thyroid: Anxiety, harsh on themselves, competing with self and others.

BACK PROBLEMS

Secondary Gain: When I need support and my back goes out people will help or understand. My partner will get off my back. Wanting to back out. (**see above)

Temporary Admission: Feeling unsupported in a relationship (work or intimate). Fear of money conditions now and or in the future.

Goal: I am supported, I am supporting.

Purpose: Is to provide support and stability.

Vice to Virtue: Strong, Balanced, Connected, Peace, Courage.

Sciatica: sexual conflict, focus on money, being hypocritical.

BRAIN

Secondary Gain: If I get overwhelmed I can freeze up, like a computer. (**see above)

Temporary Admission: I am controlling, I am anxious, I am failing at communication

Goal: I let go, I can connect.

Purpose: controls our emotional and physical body, controls bodily function, like a hologram computer.

Vice to Virtue:

See Migraine, Headache, Anxiety.

Aneurysm: Pressure internalized.

Cerebellum: Unbalanced in life.

Concussion: Too much stress, need a break.

Tremor: Depression, strong unresolved control issues.

Parkinson: Passive-aggressive, strong unresolved control issues, checking out with fear

Alzheimer's: Passive-aggressive, strong unresolved control issues, checking out hopelessly.

Tumor: Set in your own beliefs, stubborn. Refusing to change.

BONE
Secondary Gain: To receive support, (**see above).
Temporary Admission: I lack stability, I lack courage.
Goal: I am indestructible, I am strong, courage and vitality.
Purpose: To give minerals to a stressed body.
Vice to Virtue: Equal, Courage, Patience, Peace.
Break: Rebelling against masculine form or authority. Issue with time.
Osteoporosis: Not feeling strong or supported – see thyroid.

BREAST
Secondary Gain: Gives me a chance to nurture myself. (**see above).
Temporary Admission: I am controlling, I am separate. I don't trust.
Goal: To let go and connect trust.
Purpose: To allow you to connect with your internal.
Vice to Virtue: Equal, Courage, Patience, Peace
Left: Children and mothering
Right: Partners

CANCER
Secondary Gain: Safe mode, my turn, giving up. Loss of control in life. (**see above)
Temporary Admission: I am guilty, I want it to be my turn. I don't know how to get my needs met. I am controlling. I am mutated
Goal: I am connected, I am equal, I have faith. I let go of my need to control. (maybe: I want to live, I can receive, I can let go). I can change and not mutate.
Purpose: Self-preservation, external threats are too great and the need to retreat.
I let go of my need to control – Cancer's uncontrolled growth is a mirror of the losing fight.
Vice to Virtue: Connect, Courage, Equal, Unwavering, Honest
Bladder: Guilt, anxiety
Bone: Self-punishment, emotional pressure.
Breast: Worry(anxiety), conflict, repressed emotions (anger)
Colorectal: Hate, condemnation
Endocrine: Imbalance in family, work, and life.
Stomach: Revenge, hate
Kidney: Fear, childish
Leukemia: Depression, repressed anger
Liver: Anger, resentment, scarcity, starving for ...
Lung: Grief, guilt
Non-Hodgkins: Fear, depression
Pancreatic: Money conflict, no sweetness in life
Prostate: Masculinity, Fear in aging,
Reproductive: see reproductive
Skin: Integrity

CODEPENDENCY & CARETAKING BEHAVIOR

Secondary Gain: If I give more than I take - those around me will always either be indebted or need me. Maintain perceived control. Soothes my abandonment issues.

Temporary Admission: I am controlling, I am needy, I am better than. I lack boundaries, I am not aware of my feelings, I fear being abandoned or unwanted, I have low self-esteem. I'm only OK when you're OK. Fixing you relieves my anxiety.

Goal: I am willing and able to receive. I have boundaries, I am open to my feelings.

Purpose: To be needed, and or wanted.

Vice to Virtue: Equal, Peace, Patience

CONTROLLING (FEELING CONTROLLED)

Secondary Gain: If I have control over things I don't need to change. If I feel controlled I can control others in a passive-aggressive way.

Temporary Admission: I am controlling, I am separate. I don't trust.

Goal: To let go and connect trust.

Purpose: To allow you to connect with your internal. Letting go of control allows you to shift from external to internal.

Vice to Virtue: Equal, Courage, Patience, Peace

CRITICAL/ PERFECTIONISM/UNRELENTING

Secondary Gain: As long as I am better than you, I am okay and I'm loved if I am perfect. When I control I believe I subdue my anxiety.

Temporary Admission: I am hard on you and harder on myself. I am controlling, I am anxious, I am critical, I am perfect, I am wrath, I am hostility, I am impatience, I am excessive, I am pressured. I feel incompetent. I am unrelenting, inflexible.

Goal: I am loved if I am not perfect, I can trust and let go. I am competent. Free from comparing, I set my own expectations.

Purpose: The constructive aspect of control has to do with self-esteem and autonomy. We seek constructive control to succeed. The destructive aspect of control maintains control, power or superiority over others

Vice to Virtue: Competent, Humility, Equal, Diligence, Patience.

Punishing: Harsh punishment, shame, and guilt for making mistakes. Impatience, Unforgiving of yourself.

Pessimistic: Belief in Forever and Universal. I focus on the negative, exaggerated fear

CUT OFF EMOTIONS

(repressed anger, passive-aggressive)

Secondary Gain: If I don't show my emotions I am better than those who wear their emotions on their sleeves. Or, I will not get disapproval, I will be liked. It feels safe to feel superior.

Temporary Admission: I am being angry, I am rage or wrath, I am frustrating. I am passive-aggressive. I have checked out, I am fearful, etc.

Goal: If I express what I feel it is safe. I am equal, I have courage.

Purpose: The constructive purpose of expressing emotions is to get needs met, to address and resolve the negative emotion, to feel love. The destructive aspect is blaming how you feel on others, repressing emotions in our body.

Vice to Virtue: Equal, Courage, Patience, Peace.

DEPRESSION
Secondary Gain: I get attention and a break when I am depressing, I can control others by being depressing or dejected...I can control. I get to isolate and not take responsibility. Believing in the "poor me" feels good temporarily. I can see things more accurately, not falsely optimistic. (**see above)

Temporary Admission: I am depressing, I feel dejected, I am anxious, I am passive-aggressive. I am controlling. I have self-doubt. I am ruminating. If only....

Goal: I have hope, I have control, I confront my fear.

Purpose: As an evolutionary mechanism in social structures, possibly a passive-aggressive way to deal with authority and anxiety. Ruminating allows me to figure things out, by looking inwards. Failure to gain status, Fall from hierarchy.

Those experiencing periods of depressing have objective lenses more accurate than falsely optimistic people. This aids them in seeing things objectively and making changes.

Vice to Virtue: Diligence, Temperance, Courage, Balanced.

See: Anxiety, Control

DIGESTION, BOWELS, INTESTINE
Secondary Gain: Give me a break from process and assimilating. (**see above)

Temporary Admission: I feel insecure, I can't let go of things, I am afraid, combined with anger.

Goal: I am secure, I let go, I take things in. I can release the past and absorb the present.

Purpose: Digest, assimilate, process and eliminate.

Vice to Virtue: Temperance.

Anus: Power and Control.

Rectum: Self-worth, Want is my function.

Bowels: Control, flow.

Colon: Longstanding conflict, hate.

Celiac Gluten: Anxiety, depression, overreacting, trouble assimilating the hard things in life.

Diarrhea: Running away, fear, anxiety.

Constipation: Holding on.

Ulcerative Colitis: Anxiety, obsessive.

Candida: Control, blaming.

Ulcers: Anxiety, worry, revenge.

DIABETES
Secondary Gain: Wanting more sweetness. (**see above)

Temporary Admission: I am gluttonous, I am sedentary, I am hostile, I am anxious, I am negative, I am bitter, wanting to do things over.

Severely judging self and others, Disappointment and sorrow in life, Control issues

Goal: I am conscientious, I am optimistic, I am temperance, life is sweet, I want to address my feelings.

Purpose: Diabetes is a function of failed digestion of fats, proteins, and carbohydrates, not just a sugar handling problem. Ask why the body is not digesting fats, proteins, and carbs? Is the consumer eating the wrong type or too much?

Vice to Virtue: Diligence, Temperance, Kindness.

DRUG CONSUMPTION - Prescription or Street
Secondary Gain: I feel great, I can escape from reality and responsibility, I don't have to deal with (_____). Numb painful feelings, punish yourself. Give you confidence, temporary high, stress relief, and escape responsibilities
Temporary Admission: Dealing with my pain is too difficult. My hurts are too big.
Goal: All my issues can be solved, temporary and specific.
Purpose: Constructive aspect is to avoid pain because you are not ready to deal with the Emotion-Link. Destructive aspect is to cause more pain to guide you to your purpose and ask you to deal with the pain.
Vice To Virtue: Open, Courage, Diligence.
See Undisciplined, Alcohol.

EARS
Secondary Gain: I don't have to listen to what I don't want to hear, or what angers me or causes fear. (**see above)
Temporary Admission: I am in denial, It is easier to turn down the volume then to assert myself.
Goal: I am open to listening, I set healthy boundaries.
Purpose: To shut out what I don't want to hear.
Vice to Virtue: Honesty.
Middle ear: Not wanting to hear the conflict.

ELBOWS
Secondary Gain: Pushing people away gives me distance. (**see above)
Temporary Admission: I have difficulty changing directions, I am pushing people away, I have difficulty with change.
Goal: I am open to change, I set healthy boundaries.
Purpose: To give us space and direction. Movement forward and laterally.
Vice to Virtue: Open, Strong, Courage.

ENDOCRINE GLAND
Secondary Gain: When I am off-balance, I need a break. I seek and gain control. **
Temporary Admission: I am out of balance, in my family, work, play.
Goal: I have a balance.
Purpose: to regulate and balance metabolism, growth and hormone production.
Vice to Virtue: Temperance, Fair, Equal, Cooperate.
Adrenal: See adrenal.
Hypothalamus: See brain.
Pituitary: Control issues.
Pineal: Closed off.
Thymus: Giving up, exhausted, feeling like a victim.
Parathyroid: Resentment,
See also Pancreas, Reproductive, Kidney.

ENTITLEMENT - SUPERIORITY
Secondary Gain: If I am superior to you I am okay. My specialness justifies me taking more.
Temporary Admission: I am superior, I feel inferior, I am better than you, I deserve more than you. I am dominating, I am competing, I am controlling.
Goal: I am equal, I am generous. I am empathetic.
Purpose: To shut out what I don't want to hear.
Vice to Virtue: Equality, Charity, Fair.

FAILURE
Secondary Gain: If I don't make an attempt I can't fail. If I depend on someone I never have to make decisions. If I fail I can blame others and not take responsibility
Temporary Admission: I am a failure, I stupid, I can't do it as well as… I am inadequate, incompetent, helpless.
Goal: If I do the work I will get results. I can grow and change, I will learn from setbacks. I can do this.
Purpose: To lead us to success.
Vice to Virtue: Courage, Strength, Ambitious.
Dependence: I need help, passive, avoids conflict, people pleaser, no boundaries.

FINANCIAL PAIN
Secondary Gain: If I overspend I feel important and fit in. I get a dopamine response when I spend.
Temporary Admission: I am greedy, I am lazy, I am indulgent, I am impulsive, I want to fit in.
Goal: I am worthy of balanced finances. It is possible to spend less than I make. I can tithe.
Purpose: of financial pain is to direct you to the vices and pain. This connects you to the virtues.
Vice to Virtue: Charity, Fair, Balanced, Unwavering, Kindness.
See Undisciplined.

GENETIC CONDITIONS
Gain: Conflict in the family. Connect the family. Serve a purpose, and/or divine purpose. Ancestral emotions and stressful experiences passed down.
Goal: Demonstrate unconditional love.
Purpose: There is a plan and a path. Separation to healing, a higher plan.
To find purpose and meaning.
Virtue: Equality, Peace, Love.
Amyotrophic Lateral Sclerosis (ALS)
Autism
Childhood Illness
Birth Defects, Down Syndrome/Turner Syndrome
Cystic Fibrosis
Sickle Cell Anemia
Marfan Syndrome
Muscular dystrophy
Huntington's, Hemochromatosis
Retinitis Pigmentosa

GALLBLADDER
Secondary Gain: Relates to caretaking behavior, controlling and perfectionism. **
Temporary Admission: I'm being resentful, frustrating, bitter, self-sacrificing, worry. I am a victim, I am better than you. I am over competitive.
Goal: I am equal, I am peaceful.
Purpose: to store and concentrate bile, assimilating.
Vice to Virtue: Peace, Patience.
Gallstones: Concentrated resentment, hate.

GRIEF
Secondary Gain: Time to resolve, guilt, shame, fear, anger, denial,
Temporary Admission: I am guilty, It is my fault, I blame myself,
Goal: To forgive, to make things temporary and specific. Resolve, resilience. Gratitude
Purpose: To resolve. To live.
Vice to Virtue: Courage, Strength, Love, Peace, Loyal.

Hand & Fingers see Wrist

HEADACHACHES (also see Migraine)
Secondary Gain: Time to rest. I have an excuse to rest, allow me to control surroundings, the fear allows me to retreat, especially if I can't face the stress.
Temporary Admission: I am stressed(ing), I am controlling, I feel fear, I am upset (ing).
Goal: To reset, figure things out, face the touch issues.
Purpose: Rest, quite, retreat, find gratitude, balance.
Vice to Virtue: Courage, Strength, Diligence, Peace.

HEART
Secondary Gain: I can slow down. Permission to rest (**see above)
Temporary Admission: My territory being threatened. Misplaced value on money. Conflict with my love center, emotional center, Broken heart, money first, anger, my self is hardened with my thoughts. Never-ending conflict.
Goal: I have courage, I forgive, When I choose virtue I follow my heart.
Purpose: The seat of thought and love. Deliver oxygen and life to all tissues.
Vice to Virtue: Charity, Temperance.
Blood Pressure: Pressure, unresolved hurt.
Stroke: Feeling rejected, intense resistance.

HIPS
Secondary Gain: I don't have to move forward. (**see above)
Temporary Admission: I feel unstable, I have a difficult time making decisions.
Goal: I look forward to the future and direction.
Purpose: To give us steadiness and movement forward.
Vice to Virtue: Strength, Courage.
Hips Right: future and things.
Hip Left: future and family.

HYPOCHONDRIAC
Secondary Gain: When I worry about things they don't happen. People will give me attention.
Temporary Admission: I feel paranoid, I feel afraid, I exaggerate my fear to ease my mind. I am catastrophic.
Goal: I can manage illness or trauma.
Purpose: To give warning of danger.
Vice to Virtue: Peace, Balance, Courage.

INSOMNIA
Secondary Gain: See anxiety, guilt (**see above)
Temporary Admission: I feel guilty, I can't let go, I can't figure this out.
Goal: I let go, I want to know, I have gratitude.
Purpose: of sleep is to process, detox, digest and assimilate the thoughts, actions, etc. of the day.
Vice to Virtue: Balance, Diligence, Connected, Peace, Strong.
Snoring: Stuck in old patterns, Lacking flow.
Sleep Apnea: Stubborn, resentment.
Narcolepsy: Can't cope. Running away, checking out.

JAW - TMJ
Secondary Gain: I am better than you if I don't show my emotions. (**see above)
Temporary Admission: I am resentful, frustrating, Anger, Wanting to get even thoughts, Fear of expression.
Goal: I am being forgiving, I let go.
Purpose: is to breakdown and assimilate food and speaking, Expression, communication.
Vice to Virtue: Forgiveness, Patience.

KIDNEY
Secondary Gain: **see above)
Temporary Admission: I am being childish, I need control, I am critical, disappointed, or failure with life. I am afraid.
Goal: I am mature, I have pure thoughts.
Purpose: Filter blood, eliminate waste, create balance, make hormones, regulate blood pressure. The seat of temperance, energy, and wisdom. Kidneys represent exchange, give-and-take.
Vice to Virtue: Courage, Humility, Strength.
Right Kidney: Energy.
Left Kidney: Sexuality.

KNEE PAIN
Secondary Gain: **See above.
Temporary Admission: I am being inflexible, My ego and pride get in the way, I am not flexible to authority
Goal: I am flexible, I let go.
Purpose: Bring you to your knees.
Vice to Virtue: Courage, Ambitious, Kindness, Strong, Balanced, Equal.
Left Knee: feminine - undervalued, obsessive, emotional pain, insecure, low self-worth.
Right Knee: masculine – issue with time, an issue with authority, want to be right, ego.

LIVER

Secondary Gain: Being angry or aggressive protects me from danger, it is a release. (**see above)

Temporary Admission: I don't think I am getting enough, I am critical and complaining. Believe in scarcity.

Goal: I am happy, being brave. I am getting enough, I am the joy.

Purpose: to filter, detox and metabolize. Symbolizes lust.

Vice to Virtue: Charity, Temperance, Patience.

Hemorrhoids:: Pressure with deadlines, anxiety, "leave me alone."

Varicose Veins: Tension, backflow, resisting.

Jaundice: Afraid, cowardly.

Mononucleosis: exhausted, worn out, passive-aggressive.

LIVING THROUGH OTHERS - TV MEDIA CONSUMPTION

Secondary Gain: My life is okay compared to theirs. Fill the void. I'm not alone, I relate and live vicariously. Need for approval, need to be grandiose.

Temporary Admission: I have low self-esteem. I feel better when I watch other people's drama. I live through others. It is safer that way. I am boring or not ready for connecting.

Goal: I seek to do the things I am good at. I don't need approval, I don't need to be superior, I seek to connect.

Purpose: The constructive aspect is to connect with like-minded people. The destructive aspect is to envy, obsess, deflect.

Vice to Virtue: Connected, Kindness.

LUNGS

Secondary Gain: When I don't want to take in life. (**see above)

Temporary Admission: I feel grief, sadness, I am not eliminating waste, I am not taking in life, fear of suffocating.

Goal: I take in life, I release grief and sadness.

Purpose: to take in life and eliminate waste, receive the breath of life, vital capacity, elimination.

Vice to Virtue: Charity, Fair, Connected.

Bronchioles: Family conflict, intense.

Larynx: Fear of speaking your truth.

Pneumonia: Giving up, is it worth it. Deep pains unresolved.

Flu: Discord at home. A belief in the germ theory.

LYMPH

Secondary Gain: Let me rest. Allow me to recover and eliminate waste. (**see above)

Temporary Admission: I am congested, not flowing, I am hard-headed.

Goal: I am flowing, I am accepted.

Purpose: Immune response.

Vice to Virtue: Temperance, Peace, Balance.

MICROBES – VIRUS, BACTERIA, FUNGUS
Secondary Gain: Let me rest. Allow me to recover and eliminate waste.
Temporary Admission: congestion, hostility, not flowing, confusion or conflict usually family
Goal: I am balanced.
Purpose: to eliminate dead and dying cells, To restore order.
Vice to Virtue: Temperance, Peace, Balance.

MIGRAINES (see Headaches)
Secondary Gain: I have a reason to not have _____, Reason to leave me alone. **
Temporary Admission: I am being frustrated, I don't want to be pushed, or pressured, I am sexually frustrated and feel pressured or repressed.
Goal: I let go of the need for control.
Purpose: Protect you from noxious things.
Vice to Virtue: Strong, Connected, Balance.

MUSCLE CRAMPS
Secondary Gain: I don't have to move because I am afraid.
Temporary Admission: I am being afraid, feeling the tension, pressure.
Goal: I embrace my fears, I trust in the process.
Purpose: Slow you down to get nutrients to the muscle.
Vice to Virtue: Courage, Equality.
Calf Muscle: Exhaustion (see Adrenal)
Quadriceps: Anger, Frustration (see Liver)
Chest: Courage (see The Heart)
Hamstring: Stubborn, Defensive.
Foot: Fear.
Low Back: Relationship Stress.
Menstrual: Sexual Guilt, Fear.

NAUSEA/ VOMITING
Secondary Gain: Escape from fear, retreat and rest. I have an excuse to reject what it is I am rejecting.
Temporary Admission: I am rejecting, I am in denial, I am feeling disgusted(ing)
Goal: I want to accept, embrace, and take in. I want to assimilate and not judge.
Purpose: Balanced hormones for stress, survival, and sexuality. When I control blood sugar, burn protein and fat, I can react to stressors like illness or injury.
Vice to Virtue: Courage, Strength, Peace, Faith.

NECK
Secondary Gain: If shoulders are in pain I may be given a break from the burdens, someone else takes the load. Being inflexible allows me to be "right." **see above)
Temporary Admission: I am not flexible to see the other way, I am being a pain in the neck. My balance is disturbed. I am stubborn, I refuse to see the other side.
Goal:: I am balanced, I have the ability to see the other side. I am not guilty. I seek to understand, and then be understood.
Purpose: Neck represents what I see behind and besides. It represents the spiritual plane and balances with the world we move through, it is about balancing.
Vice to Virtue: Courage Ambitious Diligence Patience, Honesty, Forgiving.

PANCREAS
Secondary Gain: I don't have to fill up my tank. (**see above)
Temporary Admission: I feel angry, Judgmental, Lack of sweetness, I feel guilty, Family conflict with money. My ego gets in the way.
Goal: I have sweetness, and joy in my life. I would rather be happy than right.
Purpose: To balance digestion and absorption.
Vice to Virtue: Kindness, Peace, Unwavering.

SELF-SACRIFICE
Secondary Gain: If I focus on other people's needs first I will get love. If I fix everything around me I will be needed. Gives me a sense of purpose and value at my own expense. I do it to take me out of feeling and facing my own pain and life.
Temporary Admission: I am unable to receive; I am not good enough unless I give more. I feel guilty and selfish. Approval and attention are more important than love.
Goal: My needs are important, my feelings are important. I have physical and emotional needs. I am unconditionally loved.
Purpose: of sacrificing is spiritual and virtuous, If it is used in a passive-aggressive or manipulative manner it becomes a vice. Sacrificing and serving your purpose is the goal.
Vice to Virtue: Equal, Fair, Balanced, Connected, Kindness.

STD - Sexually Transmitted
Secondary Gain: Don't have to have sex, punishing myself. Reproduction not safe now.
Temporary Admission: I am guilty, I am dirty, I feel shame, I am lust, I am bitter, Issue with the opposite sex, I am not good enough.
Goal: I am clean.
Purpose: To balance sexuality, to move to procreation and fertility.
Vice to Virtue: Unwavering, Chastity, Honest.

SKIN CONDITIONS
Secondary Gain: A way to get away. (**see above)
Temporary Admission: Integrity, On the surface it may be inner conflict surfacing, Feeling or being irritating - Unresolved irritation, Criticism unresolved, Security and feeling unsettled or being unsettling, Wanting to getaway. Frustrating and being frustrating - unfulfilled desires.
Goal: I am eliminating waste, I am being genuine, I am not threatened.
Purpose: The skin is the largest organ in the body. It is called the integral system and provides us with integrity. The purpose of any skin condition directs us to integrity at the root.
Protects the integrity of our being, eliminating organs.
Your skin is a protective barrier to your internal.
Vice to Virtue: Integrity, Courage, Patience.
Psoriasis: Not responsible, blame, hate
Rash: Irritating, Issue with delays. Immature Way To Get Attention.
Hives: Feeling slighted.
Itching: Itching To Get Away, Want More From Life, irritating.
Dermatitis: Conflict with self.
Sun Burns: Burning Anger, blaming.
Fungus: Holding on to hurts.
Dry: Bored.
Cancer: Integrity loss, Not Secure.
Eczema: Super Sensitive, Irritating.

SHOULDER PAIN

Secondary Gain: If shoulders are in pain I may be given a break from the burdens, someone else takes the load. **see above.

Temporary Admission: I am carrying burdens that don't belong to me. I am being coward, or harsh. I give up my power.

Goal: To embrace my power and courage. Release the need to carry burdens that don't belong to me.

Purpose: Shoulders represent what carry responsibilities, family.

The right shoulder is the masculine relating to money and decisions of the future - stubborn, harsh, uncompromising.

Left shoulder feminine - undervalued, obsessive, emotional pain.

Vice to Virtue: Courage, Ambitious, Strong, Balanced.

REPRODUCTIVE ORGANS

Secondary Gains: Don't have to be intimate, my turn, Re-enforce loneliness issues, infertility. (**see above)

Temporary Admission:: Conflicted, not at peace, mistrust and intimacy issues, trauma, frigid, lust.

Goal: nurturing and nourishment, worthiness, sexuality, warmth, fertility.

Purpose: reproductive organ issues have unique characteristics and purposes: ovarian, testis, endometrial, uterus.

Vice to Virtue: Equal, Chastity, Peace, Unwavering, Honest.

Premenstrual Syndrome: Allowing Confusion To Reign. Giving Power To Outside.

Ovary Reproduction: Sexuality, Warmth: Mistrust And Intimacy Issues, Trauma, Frigid, Lust, Internal: I Am Guilty Sexually, I Fear My Sexuality.

Testis: Masculinity, and balance, strength.

Impotence: Pressure, Guilt, Conflict With Female Or Mother.

Frigidity, Low Sex Drive In Women: Pressure, Guilt with pleasure, Belief sex is bad or dirty. Conflict With Male Or Father.

Endometrial: Insecure, sadness, victim.

Prostate: Masculinity, demasculinization, fear of aging, conflict with a partner.

Uterus: Mothering, Creativity.

Cervix: Frustration, resentment.

Breast: Mothering And Worry.

Yeast Infection: Anger, Guilt, Not Releasing.

Menopause Problems: Fear not being needed or wanted. Not accepting the new chapter in life.

THYROID

Secondary Gain: When is it my turn? If I am tired or weak, I can ask for help. **

Temporary Admission: Fatigue, I feel humiliation, I feel powerless. I feel left out, I want it to be about me and do not dare ask.

Goal: It is safe to ask for my needs. I don't need to self-sacrifice.

Purpose: Metabolism, energy - produce, store, and release hormones into the bloodstream.

Vice to Virtue: Equal, Fair, Balanced, Connected, Kindness.

PHYSICAL ILLNESS: See last section (Emotion-Link)
Secondary Gain: If I am sick someone will save me. Or I can miss work, obligations, get meds to soothe the pain. It can be my turn to be cared for or waited on. False power and control. (**see above)
Temporary Admission: I have separated from my purpose.
Purpose: This illness guides me back to my wholeness.
Goal: I can get my deep needs met without illness.
Vice to Virtue: Guilt To Love.

SINUS
Secondary Gain: Create pressure, subconsciously do better under pressure.**
Temporary Admission: I am irritating, I am controlling, I want to dominate, I am depressing, I am a perfectionist/controlling.
Goal: I am tranquil, I let go.
Purpose: The irritation in the sinus mirrors back the pressure you place on others.
Vice to Virtue: Patience, Purity, Honesty, Peace, Forgiving.

STOMACH
Secondary Gain: Allows you to back out of something. (**see above)
Temporary Admission: Anxiety and Depression, Nervous, I want revenge, I worry, I can't stomach, Swallowing my anger, Independent and self-sufficient.
Goal: I am fulfilled, I forgive, I feel courage.
Purpose: Assimilate and Process.
Vice to Virtue: Temperance, Patience, Courage, Honesty, Peace, Forgiving.

UNDISCIPLINED: Self-control, Spoiled
Secondary Gain: Short-term pleasure is the goal if I can ignore the longer cost.
Temporary Admission: I lack self-control, I am acting childish, I am not accountable, I am entitled, I am better than you, I am overindulgence, I am impulsive.
Goal: I can grow up, I now have direction and purpose. I am responsible, I can tolerate pain, I can self-soothe.
Purpose: A spoiled child without limits will lack self-control; addictions and the cost bring pain to redirect you to your purpose.
Vice to Virtue: Equal, Charity, Ambitious Courage, Temperance, Humility, Integrity, Strong.
See: Addiction.

URINARY TRACT: bladder/kidney infection
Secondary Gain: A reason to not have sexual intercourse. (**see above)
Temporary Admission: I am pissed off, Conflict in the relationship. Playing games. Repressed sexual feelings, issues with order, Blaming others for your problems, Dread
Goal: I am cooperating, I am not afraid.
Purpose: Allow for natural flora to be restored.
Vice to Virtue: Peace, Honesty, Strong, Balanced, Connected, Kindness.

VICTIM: Abuse, mistrust

Secondary Gain: If someone hurts me, being a victim will provide me pity and safety. It will validate that I am bad or need to be punished.

Temporary Admission: I am untrusting, I am abusive, I am unstable, I am unwanted, I am passive, I am passive-aggressive, I am self-defeating, I am rejected, I deserve _____.

Goal: There are honest and gentle people I attract. I am peaceful.

Vice to Virtue: Peace, Courage, Patience, Honest, Forgive.

Passive Aggressive: Being late, forgetting, rebelling, stalling, procrastinating, forgetting, unreasonable, pretending to be happy, or "fine".

Manipulation: Dishonest, ghosting, seduction, mind games, withdraw.

WRIST Hands/Fingers

Secondary Gain: I don't have to deal with details, I can hold back.

Temporary Admission: I have problems giving or receiving, I am holding back.

Goal: I flow gently and simply through life.

Purpose: Represent details, giving and receiving.

Vice to Virtue: Charity, Balance.

Hands: Right hand: problem giving- **Left hand** – receive.

Fingers: details and direction.

Thumb: Insecurity, Anxiety, Guilt.

Index: stability, blaming, anger, resentment.

Middle: sex, fear and anger.

Fourth: grief and worry.

Little: family, passive aggressive.

WEIGHT GAIN - OVERWEIGHT

Secondary Gain: Protection / Barrier, Slow you down - make you uncomfortable. Avoid malnutrition, scarcity. Store toxins that are not eliminated. Energy for growth, reproduction and immune function. Inflammatory State. Directing you to your feelings

Temporary Admission: I want to numb painful feelings, I want to punish myself.

Goal: I am secure, I am lovable, I accept myself, I am safe.

Purpose: Biological obesity was rare 100 years ago; on an evolutionary level whenever scarcity or malnutrition is present humans are prone to store fat. Today we have processed foods, gut microbe (bacteria) imbalances, and estrogenic toxins of which we have the ability to influence all factors.

Vice to Virtue: Diligence, Temperance, Charity, Fair.

See Undisciplined.

DEFICIENCY	VIRTUE/VALUE	EXCESS
FEAR/COWARD	COURAGE	HARSH/RASH
PROCRASTINATE/LAZY	AMBITIOUS	UNRELENTING
INCOMPETENT	COMPETENT	PERFECTION
DEPRIVATION	TEMPERANCE	GLUTTONY
SHAME	HUMILITY	PRIDE
SELF PITY	EQUAL	SUPERIORITY
VICTIM	PEACE	ABUSIVE/PERP
RESENTMENT/VICTIM	FORGIVING	PUNITIVENESS
INSINCERE/ DISGUST	HONESTY, PURITY	TEMPTATION
PASSIVE AGGRESSIVE	PATIENCE	VIOLENT WRATH
GUILT/ UNETHICAL	INTEGRITY/JUSTICE	CORRUPTION
DENIAL	HONEST	DISHONEST
SCARCITY	CHARITY	GREED
SELF SACRIFICE	FAIR	ENTITLEMENT
DEPENDENT	STRONG	CONTROLLING
DEFECTIVE	BALANCED	GRANDIOSE
SLOTH/LAZINESS	DILIGENCE	OBSESSIVE
LUST	UNWAVERING/FAITHFUL	CORRUPTION
ABANDONED/ALIENATE	CONNECTED	DEPENDENT
INDIFFERENCE	KINDNESS	JEALOUS
OVERLY HUMBLE	BALANCE- PRIDE	VAIN
FALSELY MODEST	TRUTHFUL	BOASTFUL
DISLOYAL	LOYALTY	UNTRUSTING
POVERTY	VALUE	COMPETITION
ADDICTION	LOVE	MATERIALISM

THE SERMON ON THE MOUNT

It is fitting to end this book where it started for me - The Sermon. For any person questioning the substance of this book and workbook refer to the Sermon on the Mount/Beatitudes. It is the basis of each section of the material presented; if you do not like how I deliver it then go to the source. I know that the Sermon on the Mount answers all of our questions and guides us to resolution of all our issues. We just have to choose God (Allah, Buddha, Brahman, or Yahweh) - The Grand Purpose.

THE BEATITUDES FOR WHOLE HEALTH

"Blessed are the poor in spirit, for theirs is the kingdom of heaven."
No false gods of money, drugs, healers
Humbled by illness: in health, relationships and finance
"Blessed are they who mourn, for they shall be comforted."
Embrace pain: It has its purpose in health, relationships and finance.
"Blessed are the meek, for they shall inherit the earth."
Those who are gentle with self-control shall become prosperous in health, relationships and finance. Not just one area.
"Blessed are they who hunger and thirst for righteousness, for they shall be satisfied."
Correct thoughts or correct thinking (conscious and subconscious). See the truth in looking internal versus external
"Blessed are the merciful, for they shall obtain mercy."
Kind actions with true conviction; No judgments, blame or guilt. Forgiveness directed inwards
"Blessed are the pure of heart, for they shall see God."
Virtue over vice: free of all selfish intentions and self-seeking desires.
"Blessed are the peacemakers, for they shall be called children of God."
True prayer and forgiveness- *"Pace e amore"*
"Blessed are they who are persecuted for the sake of righteousness, for theirs is the kingdom of heaven."

Betrayal of false friends and false gods.
Betrayal of the false gods of healing.
"In my defenselessness my safety lies." *ACIM*
Unity in healing: Connection and Infinity

> *What If?... You Believe in Change.*
> *What If?... You embrace your pain.*
> *What If?....You admit your addiction.*
> *What If?... You are gentle on yourself.*
> *What If?... You start to love yourself.*
> *What If?... You stop feeling fear, guilt and shame.*
> *What If?... You no longer need the secondary gain.*
> *What If?... You choose the Virtue over the Vice.*
> *What If?... You choose to live simple.*
> *What If?... You thank <u>all</u> of your Relationships.*
> *What If?... You are guided by something Grand?*

> *"Live Grand with Purpose"*
> *MDC*

GLOSSARY:

Curing: Eliminating symptoms of illness
Magic: Witchcraft, suggesting, enchanting
Healing: Becoming whole
Miracle: Divine intervention
Virtue: Healthy moral standards and behavior
Vice: Immoral standards and behavior
Doctor: Teacher
Physician: Treating conditions
Cause: To make happen
Effect: Result or consequence of a cause
Disease: External
Illness: Internal
Separation: The division of something into parts
Unity: The coming together
Grand: Magnificent, inspiring, and larger than you
Purpose: Reason for existence, intention

ABOUT THE AUTHOR

Dr. Mark Colafranceschi is a graduate of the National College of Health Sciences. He holds a degree in Human Biology and a Doctorate of Chiropractic. Moving to the scenic mountain community of McCall, Idaho was driven by his search for and commitment to the "Emotion Link" as the basis of true patient healing and recovery by accessing nature and principles of lasting change. His extensive study and use of functional food, along with clinical nutrition (whole food supplements), minerals, and enzymes have provided countless patients with the lasting results they seek when other treatments fail. Additional studies: Homeopathic Medicine, Herbal Medicine, Allergy and Intolerance Identification and Neutralization, Relaxation, Meditation, Yoga, Guided Imagery Techniques, and Neuro-Emotional Technique.

The focus now is on the Emotion Link and Water Fasting. He developed and utilizes a unique an effective twenty-course education series for patient education and recovery. The degree of success for patient recovery is directly related to the patient's commitment to internalizing the health issues. Along with the seminar series, individual counseling with Dr. Colafranceschi on food choices, lifestyle, rest, relaxation, breathing, proper movement, supportive care, the mental/emotional aspect of health, and the mind /body connection, provides patients with lasting results as they reach their true potential in healing and wellness.

As an educator and speaker, Dr. Colafranceschi's expertise, success and unwavering commitment to nutrition and the fundamental principles of the Mind/Body Connection, is sought to educate, motivate and provide hope through his innovative approach to healthcare. Dr. Colafranceschi is an avid hiker, cross-country skier, and mountain biker, and also enjoys paddle boarding, playing hockey, pickleball, cooking, gardening, reading, and writing.

Dr. Colafranceschi believes that healthcare is universal and has no boundaries. He believes that we are all equals and there are no grey areas when it comes to the equality of our abilities to heal.

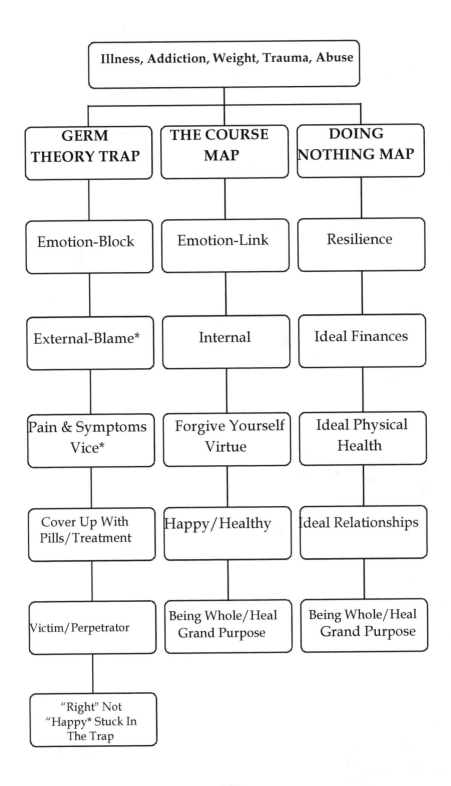

CPSIA information can be obtained
at www.ICGtesting.com
Printed in the USA
BVHW041948010720
582421BV00008B/220